LASER AND EYE SAFETY IN THE LABORATORY

Laser and Eye Safety in the Laboratory

Larryl Matthews
Gabe Garcia

New Mexico State University
Las Cruces, New Mexico

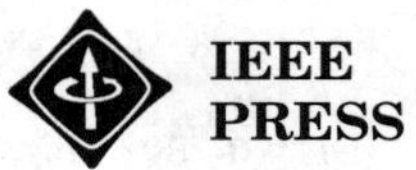

The Institute of Electrical and Electronics Engineers, Inc., New York

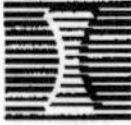

SPIE OPTICAL ENGINEERING PRESS

A Publication of SPIE—The International Society for Optical Engineering
Bellingham, Washington USA

This book may be purchased at a discount from the publisher when
ordered in bulk quantities.

Information on special prices and services for IEEE members and non-
members may be obtained by contacting:

IEEE PRESS Marketing
Attn: Special Sales
P.O. Box 1331
445 Hoes Lane
Piscataway, NJ 08855-1331
Fax: (908) 981-8062

Information on quantity discount prices from SPIE Press may be
obtained by contacting:

SPIE Press
Book Order Department
P.O. Box 10
Bellingham, WA 98227-0010
(206) 676-3290
Fax: (206) 647-1445

Printed in the United States of America
10 9 8 7 6 5 4 3 2 1

ISBN 0-7803-1037-3
IEEE Order Number: PP3863

Library of Congress Cataloging-in-Publication Data
Matthews, Larryl.
    Laser and eye safety in the laboratory / written by Larryl
Matthews and Gabe Garcia.
      p.   cm.
    Includes bibliographical references and index.
    ISBN 0-7803-1037-3
    1. Eye—Wounds and injuries—Prevention. 2. Lasers—Safety
measures. I. Garcia, Gabe. II. Title.
    [DNLM: 1. Eye Injuries—prevention & control. 2. Eye—physiology.
3. Lasers. 4. Equipment Safety. 5. Laboratories.   WW 525 M439L
1995]
RE831.M38   1995
617.7' 13—dc20
DNLM/DLC
for Library of Congress

94-27878

CIP

CONTENTS

This book is an introduction to elementary eye physiology and laser safety. Several books exist that describe eye physiology in greater detail. Other books describe lasers, laser operation, and laser safety; and a few have been written combining the laser safety and eye physiology topics. The average user of lasers in the laboratory would find these books not only difficult to read but also filled with information that is not pertinent to the safe use of lasers in the lab. Thus we undertook this writing to provide a readable, clear, concise, and informative account of the important elements of the eye and their interaction with laser light.

This material evolved over the past six years as part of the optics course taught in the Mechanical Engineering Department at New Mexico State University (NMSU). Hands-on laboratory experiments were assigned that utilized and reinforced the material covered in the lectures. Several laser safety books were assigned as supplemental course reading, but these were not written in a format that enabled engineering students to readily correlate the basic areas of eye physiology and laser safety.

This book fills that need. Each student in NMSU's optics course has read this material and has responded to the questions presented in the Questions on Laser and Eye Safety section of this book. The students were also subjected to oral questioning during the semester to review and reinforce the concepts and, incidentally, to refine the notes that ultimately resulted in the following text.

We begin with a discussion of the eye and its important elements. The presentation describes each element to provide an understanding of its function in a clear and readable form. The reader should carefully study each element to understand the overall operation of the eye and the precautions required to protect the eye against damage. References that delve deeper into the specifics of the eye are provided. A description of light sources in general, in addition to a discussion of the system of units used in this book, follows the description of the eye.

We next describe how lasers are classified, and the potential problems associated with laser operation and eye safety. The American National Standards Institute (ANSI) laser standards are listed, and a series of informative case histories illustrate the power of laser light and the damage it can inflict.

Examples and safe operating procedures should assist the reader in establishing a laboratory and work environment that are safe for staff, students, and visitors. Also included is a comprehensive set of questions that should be answered by all personnel in the lab, whether they operate the lasers or not. These personnel are ultimately responsible for their own and others' eye safety, and must be alert to any situation that appears unsafe. We suggest that the lab director keep a copy of the answers to these questions given by each lab member as a record of their understanding of the concepts presented in the book.

To accompany the example problems and assist the lab personnel with safety questions, two computer programs are provided. The first program, entitled SAFETY.BAS, answers questions about lasers and eye exposure limits. It has two parts. The first provides laser classifications and exposure limits for most common lasers used in the laboratory. The second part is a simple model of the eye and may be used to estimate the heat flux on the cornea and retina from both laser and extended object energy sources. The second program, entitled TEACH.BAS, also consists of two parts. The first part is a tutorial on basic geometric optics, while the second is a matrix-based code used to determine principal points for lenses and lens systems. Appendix B describes the programs that are listed in Appendix C. Each program is available on computer disk in executable code (.EXE) and ASCII code (.BAS) versions.

To purchase the computer disk, send \$10, name, address, and disk type (3-1/2" or 5-1/4") to:

> Professor Larryl Matthews
> Department of Mechanical Engineering
> New Mexico State University
> Las Cruces, New Mexico 88003

Finally, we have written an extensive glossary that should be helpful to first-time readers and as a future reference. The reader will also notice a feature of the book we refer to as "sound bites". These sound bites are notes, positioned in the margins, that provide a capsule view of the important ideas contained in the text.

Our purpose is to provide the reader with an informative, clear, and helpful resource to establish safe operating procedures in the lab. All lab personnel must appreciate the eye and understand how to protect it. We hope you find our presentation useful. Your comments are welcome.

> Larryl Matthews
> Gabe Garcia
> Las Cruces, New Mexico

The Eye

The human eye is a fragile yet durable and important component of our everyday existence. We depend upon sight for almost every activity that we pursue. Our eyes are exposed to wind, sand, dirt, pollution, extreme sunlight, and potentially damaging external blows (twigs, baseballs, etc.) as well as workplace hazards (photocopiers, lasers, welders, flash lamps, to name a few). Considering the array of potentially eye-damaging hazards with which we are confronted every day, it often seems remarkable that the eye can survive intact for so many years. Of course, in many instances the eye is damaged to the extent that sight is reduced or lost.

In this book we describe several aspects of the eye that should lead to a better appreciation of how it operates and how it should be protected. Elementary physiology of the eye is covered to the extent that the reader can understand the function of the major components of the eye and how damage can occur. The interaction of laser radiation with the eye is covered in some detail to allow the user to determine the potential danger and what steps should be taken to prevent damage to the eye. This book first describes the elements of the eye (refer to Figure 1) and discusses how each element can be damaged. Next, the laser–eye interactions and dangers are delineated, along with information on exposure limits and calculations. In addition, a comprehensive glossary is provided for convenience,

1

along with references that may be used to locate additional information. An extensive set of questions that thoroughly covers the reading material is included toward the end of the book, along with computer programs to aid the user in understanding the concepts presented. Any student, technician, or engineer considering working in a lab, testing, or manufacturing environment with lasers should respond to the questions. This will assist the reader in understanding the safety implications of the work upon which they are about to embark.

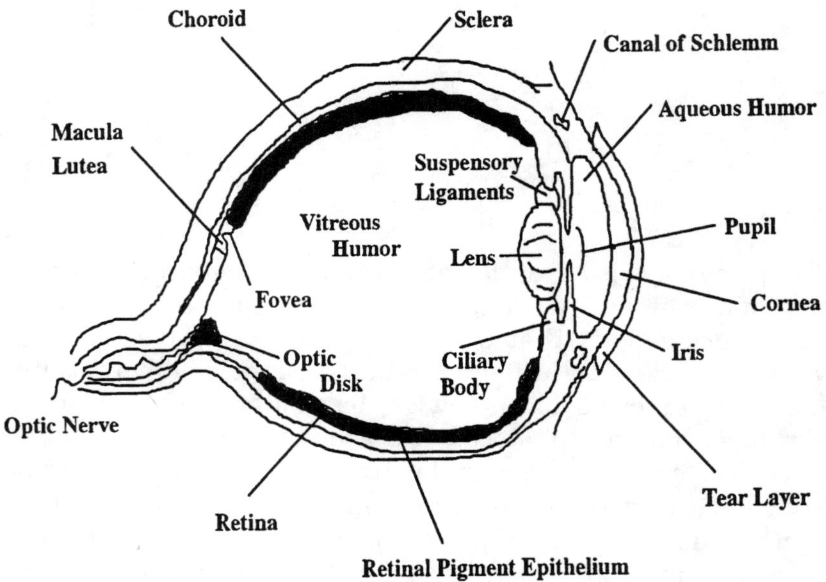

Figure 1.   Major eye elements

Cornea and Sclera

The cornea is a transparent extension of the sclera. The sclera is the white vascular part of the eye and is approximately 1 mm thick where it interfaces with the cornea. The sclera forms the roughly spherical ball that encompasses the entire eye. Metabolites and nutrients are provided by the sclera to the cornea. The connective elements between the sclera and cornea are important to the overall operation and health of the eye. These elements will be discussed in detail.

The cornea is the eye's front line of defense against environmental dangers. However, not only does the cornea help protect the eye's innermost elements; it also performs an important refractive function for the eye. If we consider the focusing components of the eye to be a simple thin lens, then we can determine its effective focal length and refractive power. Let us define the refractive power of the eye as the reciprocal of the effective focal length with the cornea supplying approximately 70% of the total.

> **The cornea provides 70% of the eye's refractive power.**

An average eye has an effective focal length of 17 mm and a refractive power of approximately 59 diopters. A *diopter* is the reciprocal of the effective focal length of the eye expressed in meters. Of the total 59 diopter power, the cornea supplies approximately 45 diopters (D, for short). The lens supplies approximately 14 D. This is due primarily to the difference in refractive index between the cornea ($n = 1.376$) and air ($n = 1.0$) as opposed to the closer match between the lens ($n = 1.406$) and the aqueous ($n = 1.336$) and vitreous ($n = 1.337$) humors. The greater refraction follows from Snell's law. Jenkins and White [5] and Hecht [3] may be reviewed for an in-depth explanation of optical concepts about which the reader needs to be refreshed. The computer programs in Appendix B, especially TEACH.BAS, can also assist in understanding these basic optical concepts.

Now let's consider the structure of the cornea. Figure 2 shows the main elements of the cornea along with the critical dimensions of each.

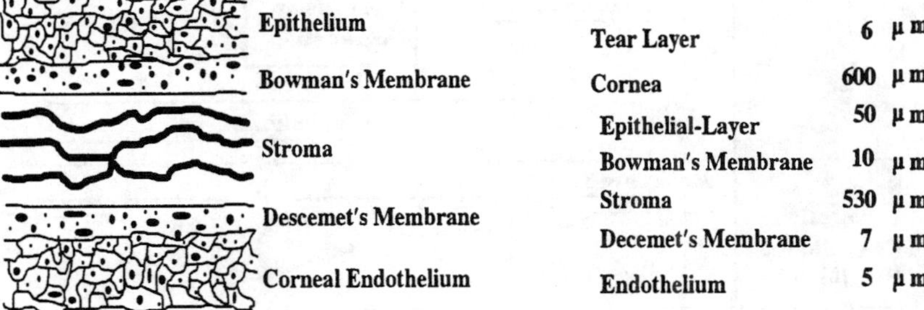

Figure 2.   Cornea structure and comparative dimensions

As can be seen in Figure 2, the main body of the cornea is the stroma, which forms a sheet of connective tissue between the outer and inner layers. The outermost layer is the corneal epithelium, and the innermost layer is the corneal endothelium. The epithelium is a stratified squamous layer that takes the brunt of most physical abuse directed toward the eye. The epithelium is protected from drying out by a 6–10 µ m thick tear layer. It has amazing recuperative powers. Undamaged epithelial cells have a typical lifetime of seven days, which attests to its high metabolic recovery rate.

> *Epithelial cells can regenerate in about 48 hours.*

Damage to the epithelium can be painful, but it is temporary because the epithelial cells can regenerate completely in a 48-hour period. In fact, the corneal epithelium can be removed completely and will grow back quickly, although this would be extremely painful because pain fibers are located among the cells in this layer. In the laser lab, thermal radiation can damage the cornea unless proper safeguards are used.

Figures 3, 4, and 5 indicate which wavelengths of thermal radiation will adversely affect the cornea. Notice in Figure 4 that ultraviolet and far infrared thermal radiation are the main contributors to corneal problems. In Figure 3 the direct effects

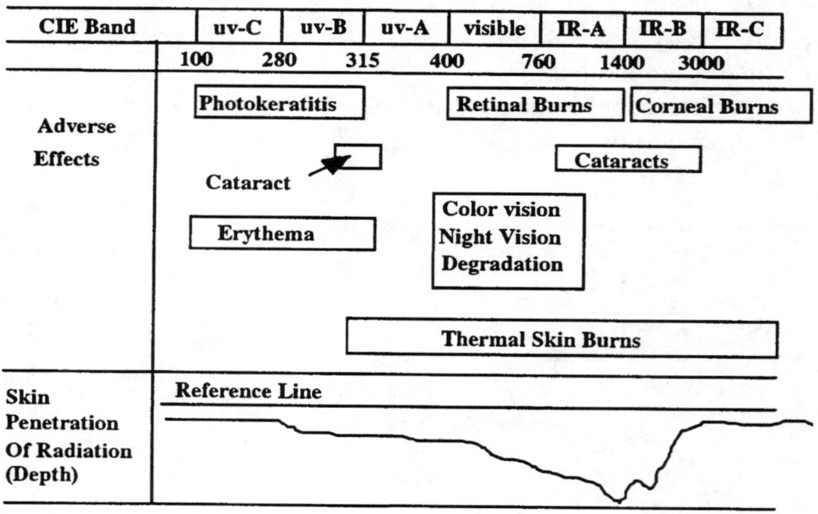

Figure 3. Spectral effects on eyes and skin (adapted from Sliney and Wolbarsht)

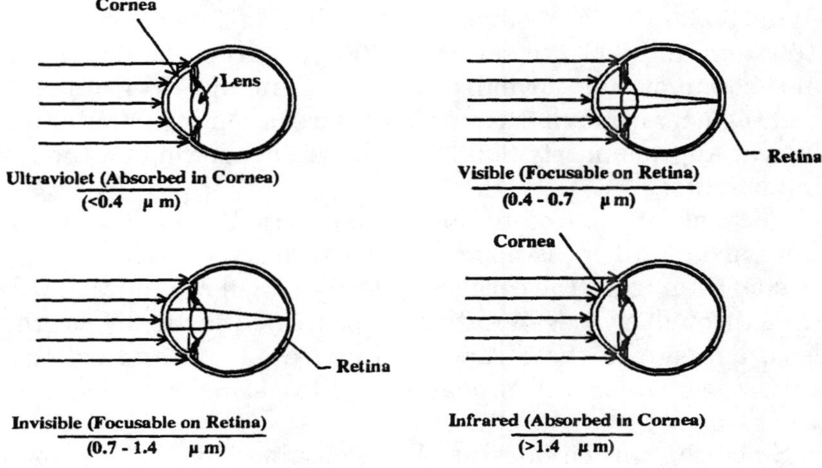

Figure 4.   Absorption and transmission of the eye

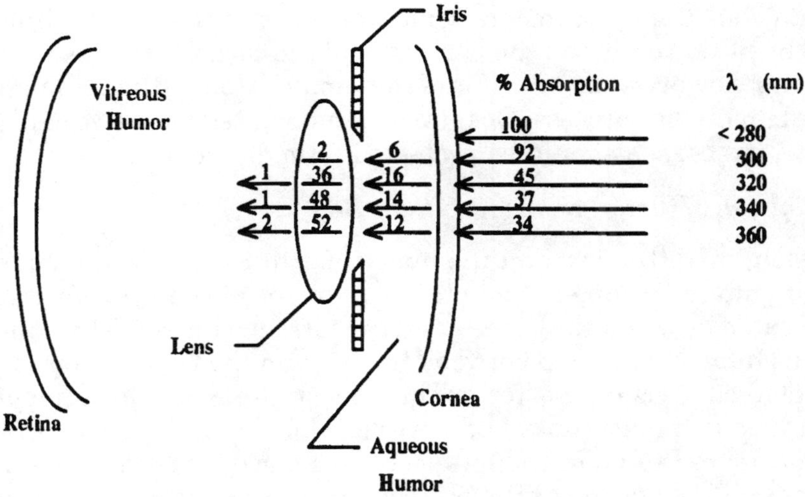

Figure 5.   UV absorption of the eye (adapted from Sliney and
Wolbarsht)

are shown. Far infrared (IR-B and IR-C) thermal radiation
causes corneal burns whereas UV-C and UV-B thermal radiation cause photokeratitis, which is similar to welder's flash or
snow blindness. Most of the lasers commonly used in optical
work are in the visible region, IR-A, IR-B, or IR-C. The most
used laser is the helium–neon variety, which operates primar-

ily at 632.8 nm. A neodydium (Nd):YAG laser can operate at 1064 nm and a CO_2 laser at 10,600 nm. Argon ion lasers are also common and normally operate in the 450–514 nm spectral region, although excimer lasers are becoming popular and lase at approximately 300 nm or lower, depending on the lasing medium.

Corneal burns, due to absorption of IR-B and IR-C radiation, are manifest as opacity or surface irregularities in the tissue. Damage to the corneal epithelium will repair itself with time through cell regeneration, as described earlier. Nevertheless, damage to the stroma can cause edema and collagen shrinkage, which will probably lead to permanent vision impairment.

Since the cornea does not have any blood vessels, it must rely on indirect ways to receive nutrition, metabolites, proteins, amino acids, and so on. Oxygen and carbon dioxide are transferred in small quantities directly to the cornea from air. The aqueous humor transfers some nutrients to the endothelium. The blood vessels on the periphery of the cornea provide nutrients; however, the transfer of nutrients through the stroma is an inefficient process. Despite its amazing regenerative capacity, the cornea should be protected from damage.

Aqueous Humor, Iris, and Ciliary Body

Along with the iris and the lens (refer to Figure 1), the aqueous humor occupies the anterior segment of the eye, which is located between the cornea and the vitreous humor. The aqueous humor contained between the iris and the lens fills what is referred to as the posterior chamber of the anterior segment. Aqueous humor contained between the iris and the cornea is considered to be in the anterior chamber of the anterior segment. The aqueous humor is mostly water; however, it contains crucial nutrients and metabolites necessary for the healthy maintenance of the lens and cornea. This is a necessary function because the lens and cornea are avascular (do not contain blood vessels) and receive important nutrients from the aqueous humor. Another important feature of the aqueous humor is its role as a heat exchanger and particle disposal for the anterior segment.

The aqueous humor absorbs IR-B and IR-C radiation, thus

protecting the lens and the posterior segment of the eye. Since the aqueous humor actually flows through the eye, it carries away small amounts of heat and any particles that may have been shed by the iris, cornea, lens, or ciliary body. The ciliary body is composed primarily of the ciliary muscle, corneal stroma (which is where the cornea connects to the rest of the eye), and the epithelium. It is this ciliary body that secretes the aqueous; in other words, the aqueous is supplied to the eye by the ciliary body. The inflow of aqueous into the eye through the ciliary body occurs between the lens and the iris (posterior chamber). Then the aqueous flows through the pupil into the anterior chamber and then through the trabecular meshwork to the canal of Schlemm where it exits the eye. The trabecular meshwork is a loose arrangement of cells, fiber, and tissue made up from the sclera, iris, Descemet's membrane, and the endothelium.

> *Restrictive aqueous flow leads to increased pressure and the possibility of developing glaucoma.*

Obviously, any restriction of aqueous flow through the eye will be detrimental to the entire organ. This is also true if the aqueous humor absorbs a large amount of energy and overheats. Restriction of aqueous flow may be gradual, primarily due to age, or can occur quickly, due to trauma (a blow of some sort to the eye). In any event the immediate result is an increase in internal pressure, which can lead to a serious eye condition referred to as glaucoma. Glaucoma occurs mainly due to pressure buildup in the eye that restricts blood flow and results in retinal atrophy (deterioration of the retina) that can lead to loss of sight. Therefore, one must always protect the eye from potentially damaging blows and submit regularly to glaucoma tests.

> *The iris is the aperture stop of the eye. It helps regulate the level of power that impinges on the retina.*

Before moving on to a discussion of the lens, a few words regarding the iris are appropriate. The iris is the aperture stop of the eye; it regulates the amount of energy that the lens focuses on the retina. As a consequence, the iris is the light regulator of the eye. It must be capable of responding quickly to any sudden increase in lighting and then be able to readjust when the light level diminishes. Although the iris might take a second or so to open when the lights go out, it can constrict within about 20 ms when exposed to any bright light source. The iris, of course, controls the size of the pupil. A completely dark-adapted eye will have a pupil diameter of approximately 7 mm, while a constricted pupil will have a diameter of approximately 2 mm. Light-gathering power changes as a function of area that represents a change in retinal illumination of over an order of magnitude. It is interesting to note that even though the iris is dark in color, it does not absorb strongly in the near infrared spectrum (IR-A). This means that laser radiation in the wavelength range of 0.7 to 1.4 μ m can be passed by the lens and focused on the retina. This poses a particular problem since the eye will not blink when exposed to such radiation. Light sources that emit in the IR-A range must be carefully used even at low-power levels due to this characteristic: they may be focused on the retina and yet not evoke a blink response.

> *A dark-adapted eye will have a pupil size of about 7 mm. A daylight-adapted eye will have a pupil size of about 2 mm.*

Lens

As mentioned earlier, the lens and the cornea are the major elements involved in focusing an image of an object on the retina. Figure 6 is a simplified drawing of a lens and a lens

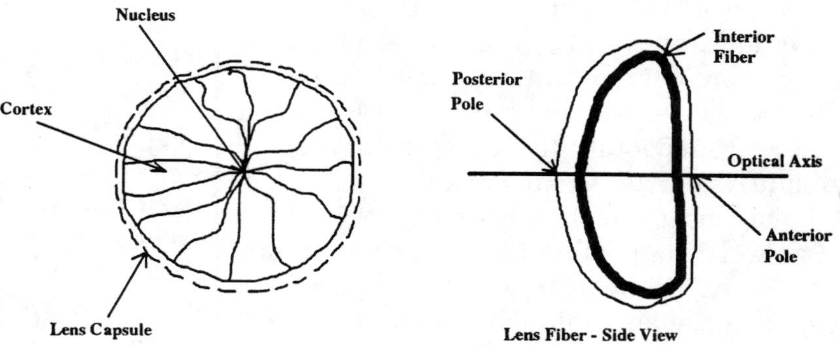

Figure 6.   The lens

fiber. The indices of refraction vary from 1.406 at the inner core to 1.386 at the cortex. These refractive variations are due to physical variations within the lens that is not homogenous. The focusing effect of the lens is strongly affected by such variations.

Although the lens provides only 30% of the refractive power of the eye, it is essential for bringing objects near and far into clear focus. This is achieved through a process known as accommodation, which means that the lens is capable of changing shape slightly, thereby changing the focal length. Accommodation is facilitated by the lens structure, transparent, pliable fibers, capable of changing shape when the suspensory ligaments, and ciliary muscles work to put the lens under tension. Note, in Figure 6, that a lens fiber is fatter on the posterior side of the lens (on the side closest to the retina) than on the anterior side.

In Figure 6, note the layered appearance of the lens and arrangement of the fibers that appear to meet at the nucleus. The lens continues to grow throughout life by adding new fibers to the outer layers (growing to over 20,000 layers!) and compressing the inner layers into a smaller and smaller volume. The lens capsule stays approximately the same size, rendering the lens more compact, harder, and less pliable.

> *The lens will gradually lose its accommodating ability as it gets older.*

Reduction of pliability of the lens causes a loss of accommodation, called presbyopia, and hence a reduction in the ability of the eye to focus on near objects. As we get older, our ability to focus on near objects becomes decreased, leading to the need for bifocals.

Potential danger to the lens results primarily from absorption of UV-A and IR-A thermal radiation. The cornea filters out lower and higher wavelengths. The lens absorption of UV-A radiation is approximately five times greater than the cornea. Actually, the precise wavelength cutoffs of the cornea are closer to 293 nm and below for the UV range and 2.0 μm and above for the IR range. Between these wavelengths, the lens can be severely damaged due to selective absorption by various chemical elements in the lens, overheating of the lens, and the possible formation of cataracts. Figure 5 shows the significant amount of low-wavelength radiation that can be transmitted by the cornea and absorbed by the lens. The lens does not have recuperative capabilities like the corneal epithelium. A damaging exposure to the lens may cause changes to occur that will not become evident for years to come.

The potential for a cataract increases greatly as the lens gets older, although cataracts are possible in younger people as well. A cataract causes severe clouding of the eye and can lead to a loss of sight because it is a coagulated form of the protein found in the lens. This opaque substance makes the lens appear somewhat milky. Even though a cataract leads to a loss of sight, the surgical correction is straightforward and safe. Basically, the bad lens is surgically removed by making a small incision in the cornea/sclera area of the eye and an artificial lens is inserted as a replacement. The surgery is almost 100% successful and results in completely restored vision. One by-product of this operation, however, is the total loss of accommodation. Of course, in older people the original lens no longer can change focus anyway and nothing is actually lost.

> *Cataract surgery is common and highly successful.*

Posterior Segment

Ninety percent of the volume of the eye is contained in the posterior segment, and of that 90%, almost all of it is filled with the vitreous humor. Refer to Figure 1. In addition to the gelatinlike vitreous humor, the posterior segment is composed of several important parts of the eye that provide for day and night vision, visual acuity, eye metabolism, and photochemistry. These other ocular components include the retina, retinal pigment epithelium, choroid, fovea, macula lutea, and optical nerve. We will now discuss each of these components and how they relate to each other.

As mentioned, the vitreous humor occupies almost all the volume of the posterior segment. The vitreous humor is a gelatinlike substance formed primarily by collagen fibers interspersed by a few cells contained within the structure. Several important functions are fulfilled by the vitreous humor, and damage to this body can lead to serious consequences. The vitreous humor must remain transparent within the visible spectrum in order that a clear image of the object can be projected on the retina.

In addition to maintaining its clarity, the dimensional stability of the vitreous body is also important. The vitreous humor forms an interface with the lens, aqueous humor, ciliary body, and ligaments in the anterior segment, forming the all-important interface with the retina in the posterior segment of the eye. If sudden vitreous contraction occurs, especially at the retinal interface (this would occur primarily due to physical trauma), serious consequences would occur.

As one ages, the vitreous can shrink and slowly pull away from the retina. Some problems could occur as a result. But these are not nearly as serious as those resulting from a sudden contraction. Such a contraction could be due to a blow to the eye (trauma) or sudden heating of the vitreous due to a laser. In either case, blood could come in contact with the vitreous, causing it to shrink and pull part of the retina with it. This leads to retinal detachment from the retinal pigment epithelium (RPE), which can cause retinal atrophy and loss of the retinal function. Obviously, this is a serious event since it can lead to loss of sight. A detached retina can be repaired, in some cases, by using laser surgery.

Since the vitreous humor is a gelatin substance, no liquid circulates through it, and it is cooled primarily by conduction to other parts of the eye. The heat transfer path through the retina and RPE to the choroid is especially important. The choroid is the primary heat exchanger for the eye and is responsible for maintaining a steady temperature in the retina and in the RPE, in particular. The choroid is approximately 250 µ m thick and also absorbs any stray light that is not absorbed by cones or rods. It is pigmented with melanin, which is a protein that readily absorbs photons. The choroid consists of a number of large blood vessels that circulate significant amounts of blood through its spongy tissue structure. The capillaries found in the choroid are approximately three times bigger in diameter than normal capillaries in other parts of the body.

The choroid is the primary heat exchanger of the eye.

This facilitates the flow of blood through the choroid, thus acting as a temperature moderator for the eye. Blood flow in the choroid is also responsible for supplying part of the nutrients to the eye; however, this appears to be a minor function. Actually, as a heat exchanger, the engineering design of the choroid would not be considered very efficient. Of course, any damage to the choroid can adversely affect other elements of the eye.

Although each element of the eye plays an important and vital role in its functions, clearly the retina is the element of central importance. The retina is actually an extension of the brain and is capable of some "on site" processing. The eye is the only sensory organ with a piece of the brain's functions in it. The retina contains a variety of complex components that interpret and process information about the object from the image formed by the eye. The thickness of the retina is approximately 0.55 mm. To interpret the information in the image, the retina uses several million tiny photoreceptors referred to as cones and rods. Cones and rods measure a few micrometers in diameter and length and are connected to nerves that ultimately supply information to the visual cortex in the brain for final processing. Cones and rods get their names from the shape of their distal ends (pointing away from the retina). In the entire retina there are approximately 125 million rods and 6 million cones.

The rods are used for night (scotopic) vision and peripheral vision, and the cones are used for day (photopic) vision and visual acuity. Cones also interpret colors and are most useful for determining the shape and fine detail of the object. Figure 7 shows the efficiency versus wavelength of the eye for scotopic and photopic vision. Notice the shift of the curves between night and day vision. Obviously cones and rods differ in the efficiency with which they handle photons of various wavelengths.

Cones are used for most of the main visual activities such as reading and looking straight ahead. Of the 6 million cones in the retina, most of them (approximately 4 million) are in the central region along the optical axis of the eye. This central region is the fovea and macula lutea, which is responsible for most of our visual abilities. The macula lutea is free of rods and very densely packed with

> *Cones provide the visual acuity of the eye.*

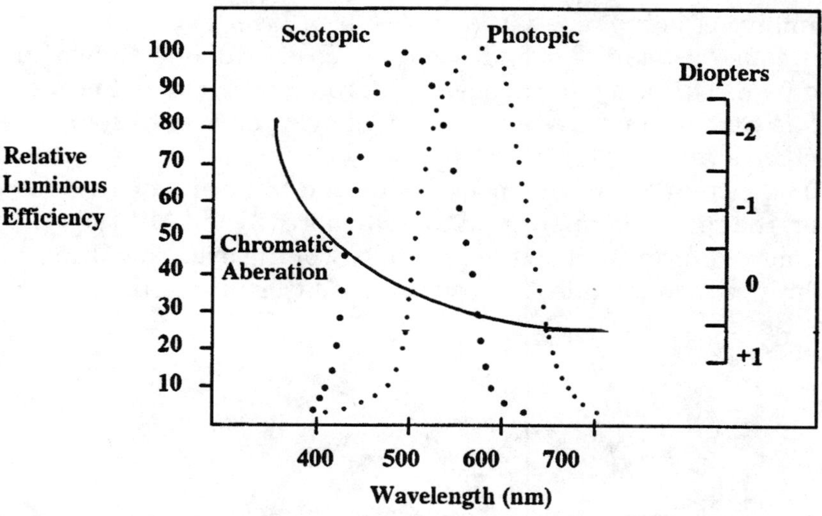

Figure 7.   Eye efficiency for night versus day vision (adapted from Sliney and Wolbarsht)

cones. The macula lutea and the fovea are approximately 3 mm and 0.3 mm in diameter, respectively.

In the region of the retina outside of the macula lutea only a few cones reside along with most of the rods. This explains why you can't read this page without moving your eyes. There aren't enough cones in the present peripheral region of your eye to interpret the words; however, the rods in this region are very sensitive. The rods can respond to as few as 100 photons in a darkened environment, but in daylight they are normally saturated and require several minutes to become active once the lights are dimmed. This is evident when you go from outside into a dark movie theater.

Both the rods and the cones are intimately intertwined with the RPE. Cones and rods are made of cellular material that sheds and regenerates daily. The RPE plays an important part of consuming and disposing the material that is shed. In addition to being the "garbage collector" of the eye, the RPE also provides necessary metabolic processes for the retina and photochemical processes as well.

As mentioned earlier, when the retina detaches from the RPE, visual processes are severely hampered. This may occur when the layer between the RPE and the choroid, called Bruch's membrane, is broken, say, as a result of laser exposure. This can cause a painful retinal lesion such as the one shown in Figure 8. This is a painful event that could be avoided if proper safety precautions are taken when using intense light sources, such as a laser.

The remainder of this book is devoted to laser safety; however, the reader is referenced to Graymore [2] and Mihran [10] for more information on the physiology of the eye. The Mihran reference also includes a discussion of laser interactions with eye tissue.

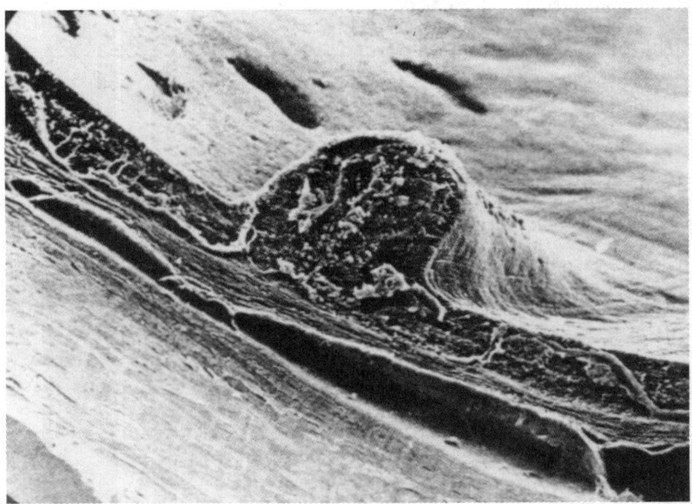

Figure 8.   Retinal lesion in a rabbit (adapted from Sliney and Wolbarsht)

LIGHT SOURCES AND UNITS

Introduction

The eye is subjected to a great number of light sources during its waking hours—many of which are potential safety hazards. These light sources come in many varieties, shapes, and sizes. Incandescent lights, photocopier lights, flash lamps, lasers, and the Sun are all excellent examples of the type of light sources to which the eye is exposed every day. Let us discuss the sources and the possible dangers that await the eye during its exposure to these light sources. We shall not describe light sources in detail, however. When more detail is needed, the reader is refered to the references at the end of this book. Our primary interest is to delineate the features of, and differences in, various light sources as they pertain to eye safety. This information is needed to fully appreciate the discussion about the basic elements of the eye and how damage can occur. If, however, you possess a good understanding of light sources and how energy propagates from them, please proceed to the discussion in the Basic Heat Transfer section.

Extended Sources

Extended sources may be considered as emitting light in all directions (or at least over a wide angle). The important property of such a source is that an imaging system, such as the eye, can only focus the light down to a finite spot, a geometrical limit. The light from extended sources cannot be focused down to a point of almost zero diameter. The geometrical limit is determined by the magnification of the lens system. The magnification of the lens system is described in a number of references. Hecht [3] and Jenkins and White [5] should be reviewed for details if the reader is not familiar with this concept. For our purposes, we need only realize that light from an extended source cannot be focused onto the back of our eye (called the retina) in a spot smaller than its diffraction limit or smaller than a spot dictated by the rules of geometrical optics. In fact, the eye is *not* diffraction limited, and the resulting image will be larger than the theoretical limit associated with diffraction as well as that determined by the magnification equations of geometrical optics. When the image size is bigger than it could be, less potential damage results because the energy is spread across a greater area. This knowledge is necessary to help us calculate the amount of energy that is absorbed from these sources when the energy is focused on the retina. The smaller the area (the smaller the spot size), the greater the energy per area. These concepts will be useful in our future discussions.

> *Extended sources cannot be focused down to as small a spot on the retina as can the light from a laser.*

Figure 9 shows an extended light source and the corresponding image. The lens concentrates the light down to a focused spot.

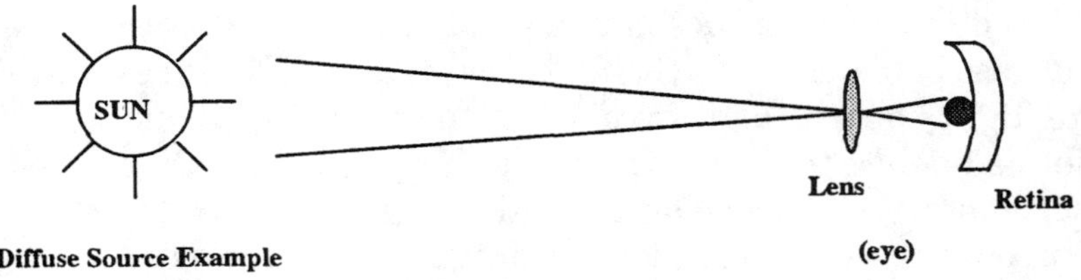

Figure 9.   Extended light source

Extended light sources such as incandescent bulbs, flash lamps, photocopier lamps, and the Sun emit light at a wide variety of wavelengths. While most of the light is emitted in the visible range of the spectrum, each source also emits light in invisible regions of the spectrum and can cause unique problems. Other sections of the book will discuss the importance and peculiar features of the wavelengths emitted by various light sources.

Although extended light sources pose less danger to the eye than collimated light sources, permanent damage can still occur if care is not taken. The Sun is an example. Viewing a partial eclipse or looking at the Sun for an extended period of time, even when your sensory receptors tell you to look away by using the mechanism of pain, can cause partial or total blindness. This blindness can be temporary or permanent. The information in this book will help you understand this situation and allow you to calculate the effects of such a light source. The Sun can also be dangerous if you are exposed to what are normally considered safe limits over a prolonged time. If you work in a solar energy facility, for example, and are continuously exposed to sunlight and do not protect your eyes, the long-range effects of infrared irradiance on the retina can be dangerous.

> *Permanent damage can occur if care is not taken.*

Working around photocopiers may also be hazardous. The lamps used in many copiers are very powerful and emit sufficient light to cause irritation to the eye. Try to never look directly into any light source such as a copier. Newer copiers are safer, but why take a chance?

Example 1 in the section entitled Laser Safety illustrates how an extended source, such as the Sun, can be focused on the retina of the eye. We suggest that the reader become familiar with this calculation and use it to determine the effects of any extended light source that might be a hazard. You can never be too careful.

Collimated Sources

The only collimated source in which we are really interested is the laser, a marvelous invention with innumerable uses. It is readily capable, however, of damaging the eye to the point of blindness and beyond. Figure 10 shows a collimated beam and the resulting image formed by a lens system, such as the eye.

> *A laser is capable of damaging the eye to the point of blindness.*

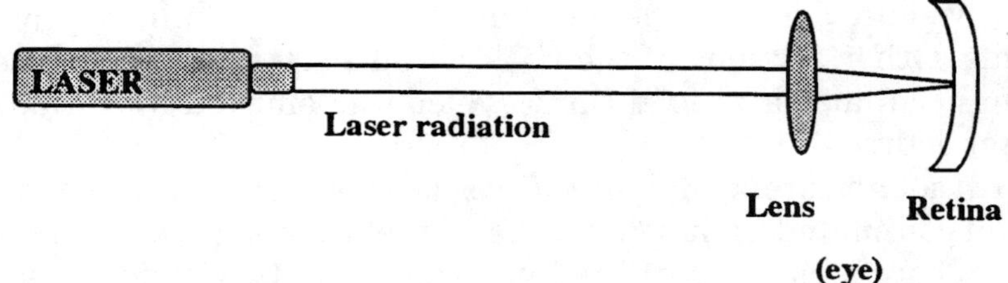

Figure 10.   Collimated light source

Unlike the light from an extended source, energy from a collimated source can be concentrated down to a very small point (many times smaller than even the image of, say, a light bulb at a distance of 10 m). The lower limit of this spot diameter is determined by the imperfections of the lens system. The absolute smallest size is dictated by the diffraction limit.

The spectral properties of laser light are unique and vastly different from light emitted from extended sources such as the Sun. Whereas the Sun emits light over a wide spectral band (covering the UV, visible, and IR spectral regions), most lasers for laboratory use emit light only over a relatively narrow band. The wavelength of the light depends on the laser and its mode of operation.

> *The light from a collimated source can be focused down to a very small point by the eye.*

Laser light also possesses unique properties of polarization, coherence, pulsed versus continuous-wave operation, and collimation. These features make the laser light unique and seldom seen in nature. Certain cosmic events demonstrate some features of lasers; however, these features are not important to our work. A short discussion of lasers follows. Several references are recommended that provide more information on lasers: Hecht [3], Jenkins and White [5], Verdeyen [17], and Yariv [18].

Properties of Lasers

As mentioned earlier, lasers possess many unique and important properties. Of these, collimation and pulsed versus continuous-wave operation are of paramount importance to eye safety. The wavelength characteristics of laser light is also important with respect to eye safety. Polarization and coherence are vital to the use of lasers in many applications; however, their effects are secondary for our needs.

We will emphasize only those properties that are important to eye safety and leave to Hecht [3], Jenkins and White [5], Verdeyen [17], and Yariv [18] the responsibility of explaining lasers in more detail.

Let's begin with a partial list of lasers that are currently available and the wavelength range that they normally emit.

The collimation and pulsed versus continuous-wave operation are important laser properties for eye safety calculations.

In most applications, lasers are used with only one wavelength coming out of the cavity at a time. Many laser designs may, however, be operated in "all-lines" mode, when necessary. This means that all of the available wavelengths are emitted simultaneously. Argon ion lasers and certain chemical lasers are often operated this way, as Table 1 indicates.

The section on collimated sources described the importance of collimated light for eye safety calculations. The significance of this property is illustrated qualitatively in Figure 10, which shows that collimated light can be focused by the eye to a very small spot. We now discuss the quantitative effects of collimated light sources.

The laser is considered to be a collimated source. It is not perfectly so, but it comes very close. In contrast, consider an ordinary flashlight. When you use it outside at night, the diameter of the light beam is several meters when projected against a wall at, say, 20 meters distant. The light beam from the flashlight diverges at a rate that would cause the power/area of the beam to drop dramatically with increased propagation distance. A laser, on the other hand, has a very small divergence angle. The divergence angle can be as small as 0.2 milliradians (mrad, that is, 0.011 degrees). Compared with the flashlight, the laser beam would be about 0.004 meters in diameter on the wall! In fact, if the laser was aimed at the moon, some 200,000 miles away, the beam diameter would only be around 50 miles.

Lasers achieve high collimation by virtue of the laser tube and the physical process associated with generating the beam. The word laser is an acronym for *l*ight *a*mplification by the

Laser Type	Wavelength (μm)	CW or Pulsed	Power (CW Lasers) or Energy (Pulsed Lasers)	Comments
Argon ion	0.457–0.514	CW	up to 25 W	0.488 μm and 0.514 μm are the most common wavelengths, water-cooled, versatile laser
HF Hydrogen–fluoride	2.7–3.0	either	up to 2 MW for CW chemical laser	mostly military uses
CO_2	9.6–10.6	either	up to 25,000 W, 500 J/pulse	military lasers far exceed commercial power levels, also several medical uses
Diode	0.67–1.55, depending on laser material	either	up to 0.1 W, 1000 W of peak power	thousands of uses, including CD players
Dye	0.3–1.0	either	up to 4 W, 100 J/pulse	military lasers far exceed commercial power levels, several uses in research labs
Excimer	0.193–0.351	pulsed	up to 2 J/pulse	
He–Cd Helium–cadmium	0.325–0.4416	CW	0.15 W	metal–vapor laser
He–Ne Helium–neon	0.543–3.392	CW	up to 0.1 W	workhorse laser in the lab, used primarily at 0.632 μm wavelength
Nd:YAG Neody-mium	1.064	either	up to 30 W, 25 J/pulse	industrial uses include welding and cutting
Ruby	0.694	pulsed	up to 2 J/pulse	first laser was a ruby laser

Table 1.   Laser List

*s*timulated *e*mission of *r*adiation. Think of a long tube filled with gas and mirrors at the end of the tube with light beams traveling back and forth between the mirrors. One mirror reflects as much light as possible, while the other mirror reflects most of the light, but does allow some light to pass. The light that gets through is what you work with in the lab.

Since the laser tube has mirrors at both ends, only photons that travel directly along the tube axis are going to get out and travel in the beam that you use in the lab. Each photon that is generated in the laser tube will, on average, bounce back and forth between the mirrors several times before it exits. This, in effect, is similar to shining your flashlight through a long (several meters long) tube. The beam from the flashlight would, in such a circumstance, be much smaller in diameter when shined on the wall as before. Of course, this is not the entire picture. In fact, it is not the most important feature of the laser that contributes to collimation.

The laser acronym refers to stimulated emission, the process that makes the device unique. The process of stimulated emission and its basis in advanced physics will not be discussed here, but is discussed in the references. The following description of the process will, however, provide the information needed for our calculations.

The gas in the laser tube is charged with a very high voltage (many thousands of volts). This charge excites the electrons in the gas to higher energy states than they would normally occupy. Subsequently, electrons will return to their original energy state, in most situations, after a short time. When the electrons return to their original state they emit photons that contain the difference in energy between the electron's excited state and the original energy state. Stimulated emission occurs when electrons are excited into energy states that require they stay there longer before returning to the original lower energy state. This process is called pumping and can be achieved by a number of ways. While the electron is in the stimulated emission state, a photon can come along and "tickle" the electron, causing it to emit a photon and return to the original energy state. This emitted photon has some very interesting characteristics. It is an *absolute* clone of the photon that caused the electron to emit. The new photon has the same energy, wavelength, polarization, coherence, and direction as the first photon. This is truly a remarkable feature of lasers.

Imagine the first photon being emitted when the electrical power is applied. If the photon is emitted in a direction other than along the tube, it will simply be transmitted through the glass of the tube and be lost. If it is emitted along the tube, then it will pass through the entire length of the gas in the tube and reflect off either of the end mirrors. Chances are that the photon will pass along the tube several times before it is transmitted by the front mirror and becomes part of the lab beam. While traversing the tube along the axis, the photon causes several stimulated emissions of additional photons by electrons that are in their excited states, just waiting for someone to come along. As indicated, these new photons are exact clones of the original. They are going exactly in the same direction and have the same energy. In this way, all photons are very similar. Hence, the collimated feature of the original photon is passed on to the new photon that bounces back and forth a few times, creating its own family of cloned photons.

An important feature of lasers is the beam diameter that is approximately the diameter of the laser tube as the beam exits. Beam divergence (0.2 mrad or more) will cause the diameter to increase slightly over distance, but as we saw, the increase is small. Most beam diameters range from 1 to 3 mm while some high-powered lasers have larger diameters. CO_2 and chemical lasers, for example, are used for high-power applications (from a few watts to thousands of watts) and have much larger beam diameters.

Usually, the diameter is measured at the $1/e^2$ point. Remember that the laser tube is full of gas (or a solid, such as Nd:YAG or ruby) and the photons are emitted over the volume of the gas. The beam exits the tube having a peak intensity in its geometric center and then falls off to zero at the edges. The shape of the beam's intensity pattern is called a Gaussian surface that appears like a smooth mountain with a well-rounded peak and gently sloping tails. The quantity $1/e^2$ is mathematically equal to 0.135. Therefore, close to 90% of the beam is included in the measurement.

> *Most laser beam diameters are measured at the $1/e^2$ point.*

Pulsed and continuous operation are also important aspects of lasers. Pulsed lasers emit light during a very short time period (say, 1 to 30 nanoseconds, depending on the laser—some pulsed lasers used in spectroscopic research emit picosecond pulses). A common pulsed laser such as a Nd:YAG, for example, will emit 30 pulses a second with pulse widths of approximately 10 nanoseconds.

Pulsed lasers are designed to store energy between the emitted pulses and then emit a burst of energy over the short lifetime of the pulse. Because of this, the average power of a pulse will be much greater than the power emitted by a continuous-wave laser.

As an example, compare a 100 mW helium–neon continuous-wave laser with a single pulse from a 2 J Nd:YAG pulsed laser. Energy is defined as the amount of power generated during a period of time. Mathematically, energy is the time integral of power. For the 100 mW He–Ne laser, the energy emitted over one second is

$$0.100 \text{ W} \times 1 \text{ sec} = 0.1 \text{ J}$$

and the power is, of course, 100 mW.

The pulsed laser emits 2 J of energy in one pulse. This is 20 times the energy emitted by the He–Ne laser over one second. Assume that the pulsed laser emits the pulse over a 10 nsec period. The average power is found by dividing the energy by the pulse width,

$$2 \text{ J}/10 \times 10^{-9} \text{ sec} = 200{,}000{,}000 \text{ W}$$

or 200×10^6 watts.

This is an enormous amount of average power! Both lasers are potentially dangerous to the eye if the proper care is not taken, but the pulsed laser will burn holes in paper, walls, skin, and most organic material in its way.

Pulsed lasers present one additional problem when eye safety is considered. The high energy entering the eye causes a sudden increase in eye pressure. Think of it as a hammer hitting you or any other object. The shock of the blow will cause vibrational effects that can damage the object. This is especially true for the eye. Obviously, a pulsed laser can damage the eye severely in several ways.

Our central premise is that the eye is susceptible to serious damage caused by the effects of lasers. Basic facts about the eye, how it works and how it interacts with laser light, are included in our eye safety calculations. Pay careful attention to these concepts. You only have one set of eyes. Be sure that the environment you work in is safe for their use.

Units

Every discipline seems to have a set of units that differ, depending on their specific area. Photometry and radiometry are two such areas. Photometry is normally associated with the way light is transferred between spatial locations in the visible part of the spectrum. Radiometric units deal with the general radiant energy spectral regime.

Many inexperienced readers confuse radiant energy with nuclear energy. Television and other news media discuss many of the hazards of nuclear energy and often confuse those viewers who are not familiar with the technology. Radiant energy differs from nuclear energy by the physical mechanisms that cause the radiation to be emitted. We are not concerned with nuclear emissions in this book. This discussion is provided for readers who are not familiar with units or are unsure about the different units that appear in the literature. Those readers who are fluent in the language of units should move on to the next section.

Photometric units are based on the spectral response of an average observer (typically a younger observer). Photometric measurements are weighted by the spectral response of this average observer. Photometric units are less appealing because they are concentrated in the region of the spectrum where the eye is most sensitive. Many lasers operate outside of this region and present a serious hazard to the eye. Radiometric units are more widely used among divergent disciplines. For these reasons, we will use units closely related to the radiometric system of units. The units we use are from the classical heat transfer applications as shown in Incropera and DeWitt [4] and Siegel and Howell [14]. There are only a few minor differences between the heat transfer set and the radiometric set for our purposes. Flux, flux density, and fluence are at the heart of the differences. Table 2 shows the comparison of photometric, radiometric, and heat transfer units. The photometric unit and the radiometric unit descriptions given in Table 2 were obtained directly from the National Institute of Standards and Technology (NIST), formerly the National Bureau of Standards (NBS), Technical Note 910-2 [11]. The technical note describes each term and how it is applied.

Note that units are often an emotional subject with scientists and engineers. Each argues that one set is clearly superior to the other. We, however, encourage the reader to select the set that is most individually appropriate for your use. *The main objective is to be consistent.*

Photometric Units		Radiometric Units		Heat Transfer Units	
Quantity	*Unit*	*Quantity*	*Unit*	*Quantity*	*Unit*
luminous energy	lumen-second	radiant energy	joule	energy	joule
luminous fluence*	lux-second	radiant fluence*	J/m^2	intensity—integrated over direction and time*	J/m^2
luminous flux	lumen	radiant power (flux)	watt	power	watt
luminous intensity	candela	radiant intensity	watts per steradian (W/sr)	intensity—integrated over projected area	W/sr
luminous flux density	lumen/m²	radiant flux density	W/m^2	flux	W/m^2
illuminance	lux	irradiance	W/m^2	irradiance	W/m^2
luminous exitance	lumen/m²	radiant exitance	W/m^2	emissive power	W/m^2
luminance*	candela/m²	radiance*	$W/m^2/sr$	intensity*	$W/m^2/sr$

*Based upon projected area.

Table 2.   Units

The fluence is the flow of radiant energy across a projected area, as opposed to the actual area. The actual area is multiplied by the cosine of the angle between the surface normal and the incoming radiation to get the projected area. Mechanical engineers will recognize this concept as the intensity of the radiation integrated over direction and time to give the radiant power through the projected area. This is a quantity that is useful for considering the flow of energy through space, without having to necessarily consider the interaction of the energy with a surface.

The radiant intensity (in radiometric units) is defined as the power flowing through a solid angle. Mechanical engineers would view this concept as the intensity (in heat transfer units) integrated over the projected area. The solid angle represents a direction and "slice" of space through which energy can flow. The solid angle can also be thought of as a cone in space. The steradian (sr) is the unit for a solid angle.

The radiant exitance is the radiant power leaving the surface, hence the relationship with emissive power (in heat transfer units). The emissive power is the heat flux that emanates from the surface and flows into space. Emissive power is based upon the actual area of the surface since it is calculated from the surface conditions. As seen in Table 2, it has units of power per unit of actual area.

In heat transfer and fluid mechanics, flux normally implies the flow of energy, power, mass, momentum, or some other quantity across an area. Hence, the use of flux for area-related quantities is not direction or projected area specific. Heat flux is the flow of energy per unit time per unit area. Photometric and radiometric units refer to density in quantities related to actual area. In heat transfer and fluid mechanics, density refers to volume. This helps to highlight some of the differences.

Do not let units discourage you. The remainder of the book uses one set of heat transfer units. This set should not get in the way of helping you learn eye safety. Review the preceding discussion and refer to the books listed for more information if you need it.

Basic Heat Transfer

A basic knowledge of heat transfer is needed to understand the operation of the eye. The examples and calculations in this book will provide the user with methods for assessing the potential damage to the eye that can occur when energy is incident from lasers and other sources. These calculations will also illustrate the concepts of energy transfer in the eye.

The following overview of heat transfer is presented for those readers who are not familiar with basic heat transfer concepts and focuses on areas of importance to the analysis of the eye. Several textbooks are available to supplement this presentation. Incropera and DeWitt [4] and Siegel and Howell [14] provide complete treatments of heat transfer topics. Readers with a background in heat transfer can bypass this section.

Basic Elements of Heat Transfer

Heat transfer describes the flow of energy from one body to another over a period of time. The equations used in heat transfer are rate equations. Heat flow is considered to be an energy flow over a certain rate, or energy per unit time. The units for heat are usually given in terms of power, or watts. Remember that a watt is energy/ time, or energy rate.

We are interested in the energy rate

Heat flow is considered to be an energy flow rate, or energy per unit time.

27

associated with the laser and eye interaction. In particular, the energy rate per unit area, heat flux, is of importance to eye safety.

When the eye absorbs energy, it begins to heat up. The final temperature that the eye achieves is related to the capacity of the eye to carry the heat away and the rate that the energy is absorbed by the eye over a given area (heat flux). We will learn that the eye has several ways to carry heat away. *The effectiveness of these processes will determine whether permanent damage will occur.*

Heat transfer occurs when a temperature difference exists or when radiant energy is applied to the surface. In our situation, the radiation is applied from a laser or other energy source, and this causes elements of the eye to increase in temperature. When this temperature rises above the air temperature or the blood temperature, energy is carried away. Of course, blood can also add energy to the eye elements when the outside air temperature is cold and causes the eye to lose energy to the environment. Therefore, the eye has mechanisms that attempt to regulate its temperature and control its environment.

> *Heat transfer occurs when a temperature difference exists.*

The choroid provides the main flow of blood to the eye. Hence, it is the primary heat exchanger that is used to control the temperature of the eye. The heat transfer mechanism in this case is referred to as convection.

Convection Heat Transfer

Convection heat transfer is related to the transfer of energy via the flow of gases or liquids over a surface or through a body. It is a mechanism that you experience in your everyday life in many ways. When the cold wind blows, convection is responsible for the increased cooling that you experience. The water in your car engine flows through the engine block to keep the engine cool, which is another example of convection heat transfer. When the water flows through the radiator, it is cooled by air. The convective effect of the air removes energy from the water and adds it to the outside environment.

When you sit in your car and watch the hot air currents coming off your car hood in the middle of summer, you are watching convection heat transfer at work.

For the eye, there are several convection mechanisms at work at one time. The blood flow in the choroid helps keep the retina and other elements of the eye cool. Flow of liquids through the aqueous humor plays a minor role in keeping the lens, iris, and other elements of the eye from overheating. Air flow over the outside of the cornea also plays an important role in regulating energy flow to and from the eye. The rate at which this energy flows in and out of the eye is the ultimate regulator of how much the temperature changes in the eye, and therefore how much damage occurs.

The basic equation that describes convection heat transfer is given by

$$q = hA(\Delta T)$$

where,

$$A = \text{area, m}^2$$

$$h = \text{heat transfer coefficient, W/m}^2 - \text{K}$$

$$q = \text{heat transfer rate, W}$$

$$\Delta T = \text{temperature difference, K.}$$

The heat flux is given by
$$q'' = q/A = h(\Delta T)$$

Figure 11 shows hot air flowing over the surface of a plate. The plate is at a temperature that is lower than the air, and as a consequence, the air adds energy to the plate. The primary mode of heat transfer in this case is by convection.

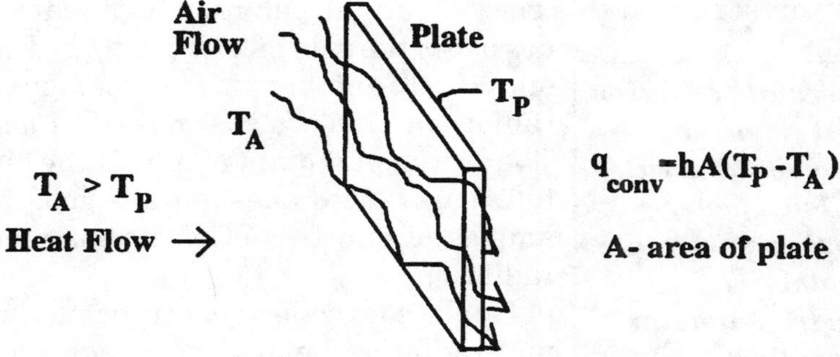

Figure 11.   Convection heat flow from hot air to a solid body

The heat transfer coefficient describes the rate at which heat is transferred from the high-temperature element to the low-temperature element. The temperature difference provides the driving force for the heat transfer to take place. It is the driving potential for the process. Without a temperature difference, no net flow of convection heat transfer will occur. The heat transfer coefficient can be considered as the slope of the heat transfer curve. It is dependent on a number of physical and thermophysical features associated with the liquid, air, or solid experiencing the heat transfer.

Some of these features include geometry, conductivity of the fluid or solid, specific heat, viscosity, and other properties. These considerations can become very complicated and are not of particular interest for this presentation. The primary interest is to understand that convection heat transfer is central to the cooling of the eye and that the safety standards established for the use and interaction of lasers with the human eye include cooling mechanisms associated with convection heat transfer.

The calculations and laser standards featured in the remainder of this book do not require any greater understanding of convection heat transfer than presented here. The laser exposure limits (ELs) calculated in the following sections include these elements, developed from experimental measurements of real eyes. However, to understand better the phenomenon of convection heat transfer, the reader is encouraged to read Incropera and DeWitt [4] and Siegel and Howell [14].

Thermal Radiation Heat Transfer

Thermal radiation heat transfer is more fundamental to the study presented in this book. Thermal radiation heat transfer describes the rate of flow of energy from one body to another via electromagnetic radiation. This is a thermal effect only. The carrier of radiant energy is the photon. Lasers and the Sun are good examples of emitters of electromagnetic radiation.

> *Thermal radiation heat transfer describes the rate of flow of energy from one body to another via electromagnetic radiation.*

Unlike convection heat transfer, thermal radiation heat transfer can occur in a vacuum. The heat arriving from the

Sun travels through the vacuum of space and warms our environment.

The photons of energy that are generated by the Sun and arrive at the earth have many different wavelengths. This is different from a laser that usually emits photons over a very narrow wavelength band. These wavelengths are normally associated with color. Human eyes can only distinguish color over a very narrow segment of the wavelengths generated by the Sun. In particular, the visible wavelengths are normally given as 0.4 µm (micrometers, one millionth of a meter) to 0.7 µm. The Sun emits radiation at wavelengths much shorter than 0.4 µm to wavelengths much greater than 0.7 µm. The sky is blue because air molecules scatter shorter-wavelength photons ("blue" photons) better than longer-wavelength photons. The Sun is very yellow or even orange when it sets in the west because the larger water and other molecules near the earth's surface scatter and absorb the blue and green wavelength photons more effectively than the longer wavelength photons.

The spectral (wavelength) distribution of the radiation emitted by the Sun is given by Planck's spectral distribution of emissive power.

$$E_{\lambda b} = \frac{2 \pi C_1}{\lambda^5 \left(e^{c_2 / \lambda T} - 1 \right)}$$

where,

$E_{\lambda b}$ = black body emissive power, $W/m^2 - \mu m$

C_1 = constant, 0.59552197×10^8 $W - \mu m^4 /(m^2 - sr)$

C_2 = constant, $14,387.69$ $\mu m - K$

T = temperature, K

λ = wavelength, μm

π = constant, 3.141592654

Planck's equation describes how much energy per unit time per unit area is emitted by a blackbody as a function of wavelength. It is based upon the absolute temperature of the emitting body given in degrees Kelvin. The spectrum emitted by the Sun is approximated by a blackbody with a temperature of 5780 K. The peak energy emitted by the Sun as a function of wavelength occurs at approximately 0.5 μm. The eye is very efficient at this wavelength. The ability of the eye to detect and focus light at this wavelength is very high. A discussion of the eye's photoreceptors and luminous efficiency were discussed in an earlier section.

Lasers do not emit photons according to Planck's equation. Verdeyen [17] can be used to understand the operation of a laser. For our purposes, the laser can be thought of as an emitter of radiation over a very narrow wavelength band and over a very narrow solid angle.

As described in the section on light sources and units, the Sun is an extended source. It emits light uniformly in all directions. A laser is considered to be a collimated source. It emits light over a very narrow angle. This angle is often described in terms of a solid angle.

A solid angle can be thought of as a 3-D measure of angle. Just as radians provide a unit measure of a 2-D angle, steradians provide a unit measure of a 3-D angle. Figure 12 shows an example of a 2-D angle, with units of radians (rad), and a solid angle, with units of steradians (sr).

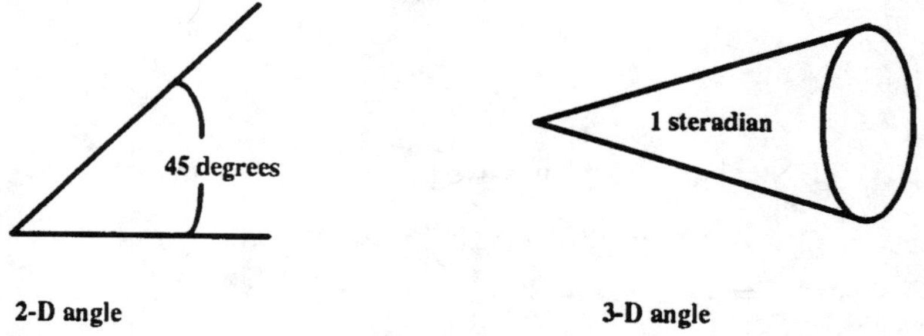

Figure 12.   Examples of 2-D and 3-D angles

A solid angle is technically defined as the area intercepted on a sphere of unit radius by a conical angle originating at the center of the sphere. For a sphere of radius R the solid angle is defined as the differential area dA on the sphere divided by the radius squared.

$$\text{solid angle} = dA/R^2$$

The solid angle occurs often when calculations are made using lasers. Even extended sources use the solid angle concept when intensities are being calculated. Radiant intensity was discussed in the section on units, and the solid angle was described as an integral part of the concept. Consult Siegel and Howell [14] and Incropera and DeWitt [4] to understand the concept of solid angle more thoroughly.

Heat Flux Calculations

Calculating the heat flux arriving on a surface (irradiance) is a central part of eye safety calculations. Estimating the heat flux at the entrance to the eye (at the cornea) is used in several of these safety calculations. Examples in the section entitled Laser Safety will utilize this knowledge.

In the section entitled Extended Sources, the ability of the eye to focus an image of the source onto the retina (Figure 9) was discussed. An extended and diffuse source, such as the Sun, emits light of equal magnitude in all directions. The heat flux calculated on a surface in one direction will be the same as that in another direction, provided that the surfaces are at the same distance and the same angle to the Sun.

Consider an imaginary sphere around the Sun at a distance of 1.5×10^{11} m. This is the approximate distance of the earth from the Sun. The emissive power of the Sun can be estimated by the following equation,

$$q'' = \sigma \, (T^4_{sun})$$

where,

σ = Stefan-Boltzmann constant, 5.67×10^{-8} W/(m^2 – K^4)

$T_{sun} = 5780$ K

This leads to q'' being 63×10^6 W/m^2. This is the emissive power at the surface of the Sun. The total power leaving the Sun can be found by multiplying the emissive power by the surface area. The diameter of the Sun is approximately 1.4×10^9 m. This provides an area of 6.1×10^{18} m^2. From this we get

$$q'' \times A_{sun} = (63 \times 10^6 \, \text{W/m}^2) \times (6.1 \times 10^{18} \, \text{m}^2) = 3.84 \times 10^{26} \, \text{W}$$

This is an enormous amount of power that our local star

generates! However, now we need to consider the area of the imaginary sphere out at the radius of the earth's orbit. With a radius of 1.5×10^{11} m, this sphere has a surface area of 2.8×10^{23} m². The power emitted from the Sun is evenly distributed over the surface of this imaginary sphere. The flux is found as

$$q'' = (3.84 \times 10^{26} \text{ W}) / (2.8 \times 10^{23} \text{ m}^2) = 1,371 \text{ W/m}^2$$

This estimated flux is very close to the actually measured solar flux at the outside of the earth's atmosphere. After passing through the atmosphere, the solar irradiance is closer to 1000 W/m² on a clear day. The same method can be used to estimate the flux striking a surface at some distance from a 100 W light bulb or from a photocopier lamp.

> *The 1 W laser produced a flux at the cornea that was 25 times greater than that necessary to burn paper, dry grass, wood, and other materials.*

From this information and knowledge of the focusing capability of the eye, you can estimate the flux on the retina. Example 1 will demonstrate this calculation.

A laser is not an extended source. It is a collimated source, or close to one. This was discussed earlier (Figure 10). Calculating the flux at the cornea is very different for a laser than for the Sun or a light bulb. The power emitted by the laser is transmitted into one direction and does not spread over a very large area as does the power emitted by the Sun. Consider a 1 W laser that emits a beam of light 1 mm in dia-meter. Remember that the power from the Sun was 3.84×10^{26} W and led to a flux of 1371 W/m² at the outside of the earth's atmosphere.

Since the laser emits the 1 W over a 1 mm diameter beam, the flux is found by dividing the power by the cross-sectional area of the beam, or

$$A_c = \pi D^2/4 = \pi \, (0.001 \text{ m})^2/4 = 7.854 \times 10^{-7} \text{ m}^2$$

$$q'' = \text{Power}/A_c = (1 \text{ W}) / (7.854 \times 10^{-7} \text{ m}^2) = 1,273,240 \text{ W/m}^2$$

The flux from the 1 W laser is much greater than the flux from the Sun when calculated for an eye on the earth because of the nature of the power distribution leaving both sources. The Sun is a diffuse source and the laser is a collimated source, which is why the laser is much more dangerous to the eye than the Sun. This does not mean that the Sun is not a potential safety hazard for the eye. It most definitely is a hazard. Care should always be taken for any potential eye hazard. The main point to keep in mind is that the laser will damage the eye much more quickly than the Sun, so special care must be taken.

The eye will also concentrate the laser beam (and the solar beam) down to a smaller spot on the retina that will cause an even higher heat flux. This has been discussed earlier in the book, *but remember these results*. Your eye safety is in your hands.

One last comment on the potential damage to the eye from a laser. In the preceding discussion, a flux of 1,273,240 W/m^2 was calculated for the exposure of the cornea to the laser beam. Using the Sun and a magnifying glass, you can burn paper, leaves, dry grass, and other objects. We have all done this experiment at one time or another. It takes approximately 20,000 W/m^2 to burn these objects. The laser applied over 60 times that much flux to the cornea, so care must be taken. Future sections of this book, especially the case histories, will shed additional light on these eye hazards.

Laser Safety

Up to this point we have spent most of our time learning about the physiology of the eye. In addition, some time was spent on eye diseases (cataracts and glaucoma) and on potential eye problems such as a lesion and retinal detachment. These are important considerations when designing a safety program for the laboratory. Now our efforts will concentrate on eye safety.

The first example is provided to explain the effects of light sources on the eye and to impress upon you the importance of laser safety. Then, the laser categories will be discussed, along with the safety features that should be followed when using the lasers. Next, several case histories of recent laser-induced eye damage will be presented with the intent of stressing the importance of following the laser safety procedures established for the lab.

Example 1 will help show how the eye focuses light from different types of sources. The light focused on the retina by the cornea and the lens causes localized heating and the potential for damage. The differences between the collimated light coming from a laser and the diffuse light coming from extended sources will be shown. The following example will help to explain these differences. Program SAFETY.BAS in Appendix B can be used to verify the results; however, delay using the program until you have carefully studied the example.

EXAMPLE 1

How will the eye focus a beam of light from a collimated source versus a beam of light from an extended source? Consider the eye to be near ideal. Use a laser (100 mW) as an example of a source that can provide a collimated beam. Let the collimated beam be 4 mm in diameter. Consider the idealized eye to be a single, positive, thin lens with an effective focal length of 17 mm. For the extended source, consider a ball 0.2 m in diameter positioned 100 m away from the eye. Also, assume that the ball is illuminated by a powerful light, reflecting power uniformly in all directions, equivalent to a 100 W light bulb.

Solution

Collimated Light

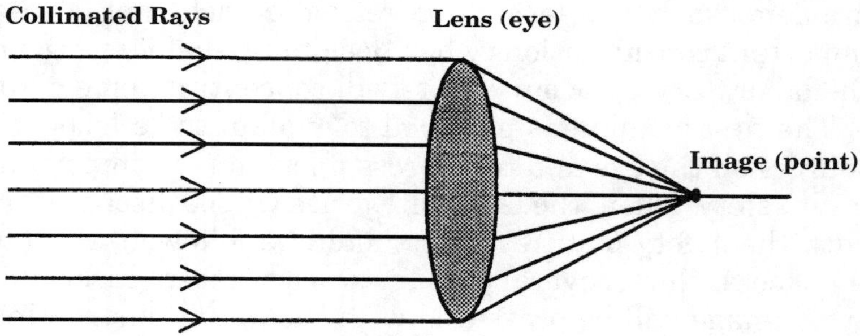

As will be considered later in more detail, the ideal eye can focus a collimated beam by as much as factor of 100,000. This is very close to the diffraction limit for a perfect lens. The laser beam will be focused on the retina, by an ideal eye, down to a diameter of 12 μm. If we consider the elements of the eye in front of the retina to be nonabsorbing (very ideal), then the power entering the eye in the 4 mm beam is still available to the retina, but covering a much smaller area. Hence, the flux, or power/area, on the retina will be enormously higher.

A laser beam entering the eye with a diameter of 4 mm and a power level of 100 mW will develop an ideal heat flux at the retina of

A_c = $(\pi/4)$ $(0.004$ m$)^2$, area of the laser beam on the cornea.

$$100 \text{ mW}/A_c \times 100,000 = \underline{796 \text{ MW/m}^2}$$

The formula is a simple but powerful one. A seemingly small power level, 100 mW, divided by the area of the beam entering the eye, A_c, and multiplied by a concentration of 100,000 leads to an *enormous* flux level on the retina.

Diffuse Reflector (or Emitter)

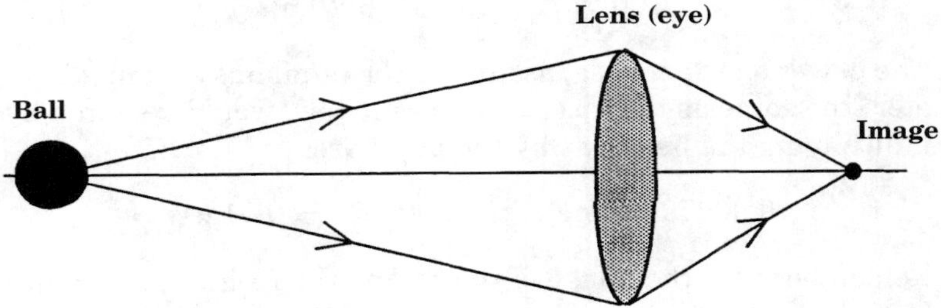

For the ball calculation, we will use the thin lens equation [3, 5].

$$1/s_o + 1/s_i = 1/f, \quad \text{Magnification} = s_i/s_o = y_i/y_o$$

where

s_o = object distance, 100 m

s_i = image distance, to be found

f = effective focal length of the eye, 0.017 m

y_i = image height on the retina, to be found

y_o = object height, 0.2 m

From the given information, magnification = -0.00017 (minified and inverted image) that provides y_i = 0.000034 m or 34 µm. This compares to the 12 µm diameter image for the collimated beam. The power/area concentrated at the retina will be considerably lower for the image from the extended source.

The formula for determining the flux on the retina due to light from the extended object is not as easy. We need to estimate the power leaving the ball that gets to the cornea. Let's assume that the ball reflects 100 W of power uniformly in all directions, similar to a light bulb. One hundred watts is much bigger than the 100 mW emitted by the laser. However, not much of the power will get to the cornea. Let's calculate the area of a sphere at the distance from the ball to the cornea.

$$A_c = 4\pi r^2, \text{ area of the sphere}$$

$$A_c = 4\pi \, (100 \text{ m})^2 = 125{,}664 \text{ m}^2$$

The power is distributed evenly over this area. The average heat flux would be the power divided by the area,

$$100 \text{ W}/A_c = 0.000796 \text{ W/m}^2$$

The power on the cornea, assuming the pupil has a 4 mm diameter (the same as the laser beam diameter), would be found by multiplying the heat flux by the pupil area,

$$0.000796 \text{ W/m}^2 \text{ x } \pi/4(0.004 \text{ m})^2 = 0.01 \text{ }\mu\text{W}$$

Remember that the image of the ball on the retina had a diameter of 34 μm. The area of the image is 0.9×10^{-9} m^2. Therefore, the heat flux on the retina due to the ball would be the power divided by the area,

$$0.01 \text{ }\mu\text{W}/0.9 \times 10^{-9} \text{ m}^2 = 11.1 \text{ W/m}^2$$

Compare this flux to the flux created by the laser beam. The difference is enormous and important. A collimated beam has a greater potential for damage than an extended source.

The 4 mm diameter used for the area for the diffuse case is an average number. The pupil usually sets the size and can range from 2 to 7 or 8 mm.

The diffraction limited image (the best image physically possible) on the retina for the laser would be 2.96 μm. This would provide an even higher flux on the retina. Program SAFETY.BAS in Appendix B can calculate each of these results. Become familiar with this program.

Pretesting Laboratory Inspection

Before testing with lasers, be sure to inspect the laboratory for safety features necessary for a complete testing operation. These safety features need to follow industry standards for handling lasers, chemicals, electronics, and other fire and safety hazards.

Fire Safety

Lasers present several fire hazards. Powerful lasers (Class IV lasers) can burn wood, plastic, paper, and other items. To protect against these and other potential fire hazards, the laboratory should have fire extinguishers located at each door in the lab and near any highly combustible materials. The facility safety officer should be consulted to obtain and position the fire extinguishers in the proper locations. Every occupant of the lab should attend a fire safety course to learn about the proper operation of the fire extinguishers and to gain experience in their use. Be sure to have the safety officer place the fire extinguishers on the periodic inspection list. Fire extinguishers are seldom needed in a properly operated lab; however, when they are required, properly maintained and operated extinguishers can save equipment and lives.

Chemical Safety

Some lasers and laser systems require the use of chemicals. It is the lab director's responsibility to identify these chemicals and determine their potential for damage to equipment and personnel. A chemical safe locker should be located in the lab for those chemicals that present serious hazards. Be sure to keep a list of the chemicals and when they are used. This will help control the use of the chemicals and provide a useful inventory for buying replacements. Keep a check-out list with the locker and the name of the responsible person to contact if the need arises. The safety officer can help you with OSHA rules concerning the safe use and storage of chemicals.

Safety Signs, Safety Lights, Safe and Clean Lab

Make sure that each exit is properly marked and never blocked. Do not store boxes or other items in front of any lab exit. Laser shipping crates and boxes should be stored in a separate room for safe keeping and safe lab operation. Install laser safety signs on every exit. These signs should be on both sides of the door to alert all visitors about the types of lasers and potential hazards that exist in the lab. Install interlocks on doors that could cause problems with people entering the lab and being exposed to laser radiation. These interlocks should shut down the laser, close shutters, or perform some other operation to assure the safety of the lab users and visitors. Be sure to install a red warning light outside each door to indicate that the lasers are in use. Emergency phone numbers should also be placed on the doors for users and visitors to have when needed. Examples of safety signs are given in the Safety Signs and Labels section of this book.

Eye Protection

Eye protection should be provided near each laser station. The goggles need to be readily visible. A sign above the goggle station should clearly indicate their presence and their operating wavelength range. Each set of goggles should be clearly marked for the laser that they accompany. Any visitor should be required to use goggles whenever there is a chance that exposure to stray beams can occur.

Lab Rules

Laboratory rules should be placed in several locations central to each laser station. These rules should be written in large type and located for all to see. Be sure to include each of the items on the Safety Procedures list given near the end of this book. Place someone in charge of the lab at all times. This individual must be responsible for making sure that everyone involved with the lab adheres to all safety rules. This is a very important responsibility. Be sure that the responsible individual thoroughly understands every part of this book and is capable of testing other users on its contents.

Safety Labels

Label each laser with information on its use. The required label provided by the manufacturer lists only those items that are required by safety standards. You should also point out the location of safety goggles, laser safety checklist, person in charge of the laser station, and a brief list of potential hazards. This additional information can be located on the power supply if the laser is too small to take a label. This precaution may seem unnecessary; however, not all users are going to remember the safety rules and the implications of not following them. The case histories presented later will demonstrate that even laser experts can get lazy and put themselves and anyone around them in potential danger. The *Laser Safety Guide* [9] published by the Laser Institute of America is a useful reference.

Beam Blocks, Neutral Density (ND) Filters

One of the most important ways to operate a laser system safely, especially during alignment is to reduce the beam power to a safe level and to provide beam blocks to keep unsafe beams from leaving the optical table. A Class II laser beam is a safe level for visible lasers. Be sure to have both ND filters and holders for the filters readily available for use. In many cases, operators will not use filters because they are "out of reach" and a hassle to put into place. The easier you make it for the operators to follow safe procedures, the safer the lab will be. Power meters are also an important part of the lab. When in doubt, the user should measure the laser beam power and make sure that the level is safe.

Beam blocks are another important element of a safe operating lab. Cardboard can be very useful for blocking stray beams and preventing them from leaving the optical table. Beam blocks also protect the users and any bystanders that may be watching. Be sure to keep plenty of beam block material readily available, along with holders for the material. Our lab experience has shown that this material will be used when it is easily accessible, but it will not be used when the laser operator has to go out of the way to put the blocks into place.

Electrical Shock

Electrical shock is also a serious concern when using lasers. A laser uses very high voltages to ionize the gas in the laser tube, or across the solid material used in most pulsed lasers. These voltage levels can reach many thousand volts. The cover of a laser should never be removed unless absolutely necessary, and then only by a qualified technician. Electrical shock can also occur when liquids come in contact with the voltage source and humans. For this reason it is important to keep food and drink out of the lab. Be sure to label each laser with an electrical shock warning and place a warning on your safety list for all to see.

Inspect your lab carefully before placing lasers into use. Make sure that all the necessary safety features are in place when operation begins. Check the state of your lab continually to be sure that the necessary precautions stay in place at all times. It is very easy to become lax after a prolonged period of accident-free operation. This is when the potential for accidents are most likely to occur. Have refresher courses for the lab operators on a periodic basis. Visual demonstrations can be used to show the power of the lasers for damage and to drive home the need for safety. If you have a Class IV laser, take some paper, plastic, wood, or even a hot dog and demonstrate the capability of the laser to damage skin and the eye. A safe lab environment and a safety-educated operating crew provide for the best protection against laser hazards. Do not let your guard down. You are the last person to want to explain to a parent, wife, friend, or university president why someone lost sight in one eye.

> *A safe lab environment and a safety-educated operating crew provide for the best protection against laser hazards.*

Laser Classification

Lasers have been traditionally classified by placing them into one of four categories. These categories cover the range from totally safe lasers to lasers that can damage the eye and burn skin.

Our focus is on eye safety. We do not present additional information on skin hazards. Skin hazards are a real concern to your safety; however, if you keep the system free of eye safety problems, then the skin will also be protected. Our belief is that every optical system should be operated from a position of knowledge and respect. *Whenever possible, the system should be isolated from human interaction by providing beam blocks, interlocks and other safety systems.* Refer to the

> *Always reduce the power of the beam to a safe level during alignment.*

Safety Procedures section for a brief listing of safety measures that should be observed when using lasers.

When aligning the optical system, it is unnecessary to be exposed to potential hazards. Always reduce the power of the beam to a safe level during alignment. Class I or Class II (for visible lasers) power and energy levels are sufficient for most aligning procedures. Your eye and video camera are sensitive detectors. Do not saturate them. Damage will occur unless care is taken.

When a system and lab experiment are properly designed, hazards to the eyes and skin can be kept to a minimum. Concentrate on designing a safe system and experiment for the eyes, and the potential skin hazards will take care of themselves.

Design control measures, when appropriate, that exceed minimum requirements.

We will mention ANSI [1] recommendations for control measures to be used with each class of laser. Another useful reference is the *Laser Safety Guide* [9] developed by the Laser Institute of America. We will not strongly stress minimum control recommendations or requirements, which could lead to a blind following of minimum requirements. With the knowledge of the eye that you now possess and the laser safety guidelines that you are about to learn, carefully review the safety needs for your situation. *Take control of your safety needs. Design control measures that exceed the minimum requirements when called for.* If you understand your system and the consequences of its operation, then you will respect its potential and provide a safe workplace for you and your associates.

Always develop and use a safety checklist for the lab. The list should include any potential danger specific to your lab. It should also require that certain precautions be taken before the laser system is allowed to be turned on. The operator and the safety engineer should sign off on this list each time. A sample list is provided here as an example of one type of list. Be sure to perform an occasional audit of the lab to be sure that all safety procedures are being followed. Refer to the Safety Procedures section of this book for a short list of areas to consider. The lab safety procedures should always be located in the lab for visitors and operators to see and use.

Safety Checklist

Run# _____________ Test Title _________________________________

Authorization_________________ Operator _______________

Start Time ___________ Date ___________ End Time _________

	Safety Checks	*Check*
1.	Access doors are closed.	_______
2.	External laser status sign is set to *In Operation* and warning light is on.	_______
3.	Safety goggles are in use (make sure goggles match laser wavelength).	_______
4.	All operators are qualified (passed safety exam and operations exam on the laser).	_______
5.	Light path is enclosed, beam blocks are in place.	_______
6.	All personnel are aware of pending start-up.	_______
7.	ND filters are in place to reduce initial beam strength to Class II status.	_______
8.	Experiment is set up and ready for the laser beam.	_______
9.	No Class III or Class IV beams leave the table.	_______

10. Make sure laser shutter is closed. ______

11. Check external shutter for position
and operation. ______

12. External shutter is closed. ______

Start-up

Specific to type of laser being used. Consult the operation manual and the manufacturer for proper operation of the laser and its associated components.

Operation

Also specific to the type of laser being used. This may include specific areas of operation that are peculiar to this laser system.

Shutdown

1. Close laser shutter. ______

2. Follow normal procedure for laser shut
down as required by the manufacturer. ______

3. Open lab, set laser status sign to
Out of Operation. ______

4. Finish this form (end time). ______

5. Inform safety officer of end of test. ______

Comments:

CLASS I LASER

Class I lasers, or laser systems, do not present a hazard to
eyes or skin for any wavelength or exposure time. This either
means that the laser is very low power, see Tables 3 and 4, or
that the laser is totally enclosed in a system that will not allow
the user access to it while it is running. Notice that Table 3 is
based upon power (watts) and wavelength (hence continuous-

Wavelength Range (m)	Emission Duration (s)	Class I	Class II	Class III	Class IV
Ultraviolet, 0.2–0.4	3×10^4	<0.8 x 10^{-9} W to <8 x 10^{-6} W, wavelength dependent	NA	>Class I< 0.5 W, wavelength dependent	>0.5 W
Visible, 0.4–0.55	3×10^4	<0.4 x 10^{-6} W	>Class I< 1 x 10^{-3} W	>Class II <0.5 W	
Visible and near infrared, 0.5 5–1.06	3×10^4	<0.4 x 10^{-6} W to <200 x 10^{-6} W, wavelength dependent	NA	>Class I< 0.5 W wavelength dependent	>0.5 W
Near infrared, 1.06–1.4	3×10^4	<200 x 10^{-6} W	NA		>0.5 W
Far infrared, 1.4–100	>10	<0.8 x 10^{-3} W	NA	>Class I < 0.5 W	>0.5 W

Table 3. Classification for Continuous-Wave Lasers (ANSI Z136.1-1993)

wave lasers), whereas Table 4 is based upon energy (joules) and wavelength (hence pulsed lasers). The laser in an audio compact disc player is a Class I semiconductor laser. *Note that enclosing the beam and restricting access to unwarranted personnel is one of the best ways to ensure that no laser damage to the eye or skin will occur.*

Wavelength Range (m)	Emission Duration (s)	Class I	Class III	Class IV
Ultraviolet, 0.2–0.4	$>10^{-2}$	$<24 \times 10^{-6}$ J to 7.9×10^{-3} J	>Class I <10 J/cm^2	>10 J/cm^2
Visible, 0.4–.07	10^{-9} to 0.25	$<0.2 \times 10^{-6}$ J to 2×10^{-6} J,	>Class I <32 x 10^{-3} J/cm^2	$>31 \times 10^{-3}$ J/cm^2
		$<0.25 \times 10^{-3}$ J to 1.25×10^{-3} J	>Class I <10 J/cm^2	>10 J/cm^2
Near infrared, 0.7–1.06	10^{-9} to 0.25	$<0.2 \times 10^{-6}$ to 2×10^{-6} J,	>Class I <31 x 10^{-3} J/cm^2	$>31 \times 10^{-3}$ J/cm^2
		$<0.25 \times 10^{-3}$ to 1.25×10^{-3} J	>Class I <10 J/cm^2	>10 J/cm^2
1.06–1.4	10^{-9} to 0.25	$<2 \times 10^{-6}$ J,	>Class I <10 J/cm^2	>10 J/cm^2
		$< 80 \times 10^{-6}$ J	>Class I <10 J/cm^2	>10 J/cm^2
Far infrared, 1.4–100	10^{-9} to 0.25	$<10 \times 10^{-3}$ J,	>Class I <10 J/cm^2	>10 J/cm^2
		<0.4 J	>Class I <10 J/cm^2	>10 J/cm^2

Table 4. Classification for Pulsed Lasers (ANSI Z136.1-1993)

CLASS II LASER

The blink response of the eye is approximately 0.25 sec, which is the key for the Class II laser classification. The eye's natural ability to protect itself by blinking is the important feature of this classification. When Class II laser radiation strikes the retina, the blink response is fast enough to protect the eye from damage. Some users take this to mean that no real problem exists with Class II laser radiation. *However, just as some people manage to damage their eyes by staring at a solar eclipse, damage can occur from a Class II laser if the user overlooks the eye's natural protection mechanisms and stares into the laser beam.* One area where this is particularly possible is in the IR-A wavelength region (see Figures 3 and 4) because the radiation is focused on the retina, but it is not readily noticed because it is out of the visible wavelength range, and hence the eye will not blink when exposed to these wavelengths. *Class II is valid only for visible wavelengths.* The primary emission line for a neodymium:YAG laser is in the IR-A region. Such a laser cannot be classified as Class II at any power level.

> *The blink response of the eye is usually taken to be 0.25 sec.*

Class III Laser

A Class III laser is not a hazard to the skin, but it is definitely a hazard to the eye. Be careful of direct beam radiation from the laser as well as reflections from specular surfaces. Radiation from this class of laser can damage the eye in a period of time that is less than the blink response for the eye and presents a problem for bystanders because of the specular reflection problem. The safe cutoff power level for a continuous-wave laser below the Class III category is 1 mW, which might seem like a

small amount of power. However, the ideal eye (diffraction limited) can concentrate a collimated beam by 100,000 times, which leads to a small spot on the retina with a corresponding high-flux level. This ability to concentrate a beam does not hold for an extended source, such as the Sun, which can be focused to a size on the retina corresponding to the thin lens formula (see [3] and [5] and Example 1 in the section entitled Laser Safety). The effective focal length of the eye, 17 mm, is used in the formula. The Class III category ranges between 1 mW and 0.5 W. When you are in a work area with a Class III laser beam in the vicinity, be sure to wear laser safety goggles that provide protection for that laser. It is a good idea to block the beam path in any areas where someone can move into the beam.

When aligning the laser beam, put a neutral density filter in the beam path and reduce its power to a Class II level. A Class III power level is not required to align the beam. For a non-visible laser, reduce the beam power to the lowest level possible for the viewing equipment being used. Remember that the attenuation of a neutral density filter is related to the following formula,

$$\text{Attenuation} = 10^{ND}$$

where ND is the filter density at the wavelength of interest.

Other safety measures should also be followed. Post laser warning signs at every access point. Never open the laser housing. Electrical shocks are a common occurrence on any high-voltage device. Lasers are no exception. Safety interlocks and master switches are also valuable. Evaluate each situation and provide the safety level necessary to protect your eyes and your associates.

CLASS IV LASER

For CW lasers this category begins at power levels above 0.5 W. When pulsed lasers are used, the rating is based upon the energy contained in the pulse and the time duration of the pulse as seen in Table 4. The time duration is especially important because short time duration pulses cause additional effects, such as sound or pressure waves in the eye, which can lead to damage. A Class IV laser will damage the eye and burn skin. Diffuse as well as specular reflections must be considered. As with Class III lasers, you should always use eye protection and cover the beam path to protect from inadvertent movements into the beam. Of course, when aligning the laser beam, reduce the power to Class II (for visible lasers) by adding neutral density filters. Another good procedure to follow when using a laser is to put the beam path at a level above the floor that is not at eye level.

> *Diffuse reflections are a safety hazard for the eye when using a Class IV laser.*

No safety precautions are too elaborate for this class of laser. Eye damage will come quick and it will be painful and permanent. Be sure to enclose the beam path whenever possible and follow all control measures.

Retinal Damage

Usually, retinal damage occurs when excessive visible and IR-A light reaches the eye. When the light is focused on the retina, it begins to heat up and raise the tissue temperature to possible dangerous levels. The ultimate temperature of the tissue depends on the spot size, power per unit area, wavelength, and the length of time the eye is exposed.

> *IR-A class radiation is focusable on the retina, but the eye will not blink to the incoming radiation.*

The laser presents an especially damaging possibility for the eye because the light coming out is highly collimated and can be focused onto the retina down to a very small spot size, which leads to very high power per unit area (referred to earlier as heat flux) values. The ability of a lens system to focus light down to a small spot depends on its imperfections and is limited at the best by diffraction. If the eye was diffraction limited, then the laser beam could be focused down to around 10 µm. It is this value that is used to set the lower Class III limit of 1 mW. The actual capability of the eye is not diffraction limited and the smallest spot that can be focused on the retina from a laser beam is probably around 50 to 100 µm.

> *The 1 mW Class III limit is based on an ideal eye.*

Figure 13 shows the actual damage threshold is closer to 9 mW for the macula lutea. These values were determined experimentally. Therefore, the 1 mW limit for Class III lasers is conservative. This information led to the Class IIIa and Class IIIb laser classification. Class IIIa is for power levels of 1 mW to approximately 9 mW.

A short discussion of Figure 13 (see Lappin [6, 7]) is warranted. These numbers were obtained using a helium-neon laser. Over 500 exposures were made in 70 eyes. Rhesus monkeys were used because of their similarities to humans. The experiment was designed to give the worst case situation by concentrating the laser light down to as small a spot on the retina as possible. Data on human eye damage shows that the rhesus monkey's eye is more sensitive to the irradiation. In some cases the difference has been as much as a factor of 2 or 3. *However*, before feeling safer about using lasers, read the following eye damage case histories taken from *Laser Focus World* (*Laser Focus* before 1989) [8] on practical laser safety and *Ophthalmology* [13].

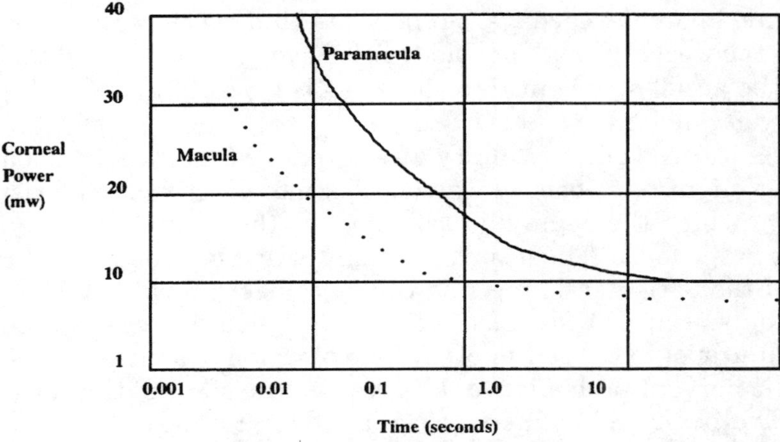

Figure 13.   Experimental values for lesions to occur

Case History 1 (*Laser Focus*, August 1977)

This is an accident victim's viewpoint of his experience.

The necessity for safety precautions with high-power lasers was forcibly brought home to me last January when I was partially blinded by a reflection from a relatively weak neodymium:YAG laser beam. Retinal damage resulted from a 6 mJ, 10 ns pulse of invisible 1064 nm radiation. *I was not wearing protective goggles* at the time, although they were available in the laboratory. As any experienced laser researcher knows, goggles not only cause tunnel vision and become fogged, they become very uncomfortable after several hours in the laboratory.

> *I was not wearing protective goggles.*

When the beam struck my eye I heard a distinct popping sound, caused by a laser-induced explosion at the back of my eyeball. My vision was obscured almost immediately by streams of blood floating in the vitreous humor, and by what appeared to be particulate matter suspended in the vitreous humor. It was like viewing the world through a round fishbowl full of glycerol into which a quart of blood and a handful of black pepper have been partially mixed. There was local pain within a few minutes of the accident, but it did not become excruciating. The most immediate response after such an accident is horror. As a Vietnam War Veteran, I have seen several terrible scenes of human carnage, but none affected me more than viewing the world through my blood-filled eyeball. In the aftermath of the accident I went into shock, as is typical in personal injury accidents.

As it turns out, my injury was severe but not nearly as bad as it might have been. I was not looking directly at the prism from which the beam had reflected, so the retinal damage is not in the fovea. The beam struck my retina between the fovea and the optic nerve, missing the optic nerve by about 3 mm. Had the focused beam struck the fovea, I would have sustained a blind spot in the center of my field of vision. Had it struck the optic nerve, I probably would have lost the sight of that eye.

The beam did strike so close to the optic nerve, however, that it severed nerve fiber bundles radiating from the optic nerve. This has resulted in a crescent-shaped blind spot many times the size of the lesion. The effect of the large blind area is much like having a finger placed over one's field of vision. Also, I still have numerous floating objects in the field of view on my damaged eye, although the blood streamers have disappeared. These "floaters" are more a daily hindrance than the blind areas, because the brain tries to integrate out the blind area when the undamaged eye is open. There is also recurrent pain in the eye, especially when I have been reading too long or when I get tired.

> *I still have numerous floating objects in the field of view on my eye, although the blood streamers have disappeared.*

The moral of all this is to be careful and to wear protective goggles when using high-power lasers. The temporary discomfort is far less than the permanent discomfort of eye damage. The type of reflected beam that injured me also is produced by the polarizers used in Q-switches, by intracavity diffraction gratings, and by all beam splitters or polarizers used in optical chains.

Case History 2 (*Laser Focus*, March 1982)

As I read my November issue of *Laser Focus*, I took note of the eye injury report, curious about the particulars of this novel accident. Even though I have been working with lasers for five years in the presence of many of the same hazards pointed to in the article, I didn't think while reading it, "This could happen to me! But it did."

On January 22, 1982, I spent several hours aligning a low-power, frequency-doubled Nd:YAG beam through a dye laser set-up. In order to see the 532 nm pump beam propagation *I was not wearing goggles*. I had also removed a beam block intended to absorb a Brewster's angle reflection to observe end pumping of an amplifier cell. The green power was increased to determine the extent of dye lasing without replacing the beam block. I did not put on goggles. While placing a power meter at the dye laser output I leaned over the uncovered amplifier and caught a reflection in my right eye. Because I was in continuous motion looking at the meter and not the beam, I doubt that more than one 10 to 15 ns pulse of approximately 20 mJ was focused onto the fovea. While I do remember seeing a green flash, there was no pain. I was not immediately aware of any significant eye damage. It wasn't until I shut the lasers off and returned to my desk to record the day's activity that I realized I had a blind spot comparable to a camera flash, but only in my right eye. It was almost 5:00 P.M. on a Friday, and I didn't report the incident because I couldn't believe that any serious damage was done.

By Saturday afternoon I knew I had a problem. Monday the 25th I notified our safety division and started my visits to an ophthalmologist. The initial examination supported the probability of permanent damage, although hemorrhaging in the affected area obstructed detail. By the end of the first week, peripheral vision around the spot was observed to be on the right side of the macula (that corresponds to a blind spot slightly off center left). I was encouraged and felt fortunate, considering the negative potential of this careless mistake. But by week two, peripheral vision had declined. Distortion (curving) of resolution around the spot became more noticeable due to additional blood pooling under the retina. If this hemorrhaging were to persist, laser cauterization would be necessary. But for now, "treatment" consists of waiting, observing, and photographing.

Although recovery has not been straightforward, and my vision may get worse before it gets better, I still feel lucky in that one eye totally escaped injury. So while reading was difficult at first, my daily life has remained largely unaffected because the brain and stereo vision compensate the anomaly.

> *Safety deserves your thoughtful consideration now, before your accident.*

But more important than the actual event is the idea that this incident could have been avoided. Don't let it happen to you or a co-worker. Take time to assess safety conditions, and do it again in six months or a year; additional hazards arise in an ever-changing research environment. Safety deserves your thoughtful consideration, now, before *your* accident. If even one other injury can be prevented by publication of this accident account, then more positive than negative outcome may result from the mistake.

Case History 3 (*Laser Focus*, November 1981)

A Naval Research Laboratory chemist who was struck in the eye with a laser beam this summer is still suffering from the injury. The victim, who requested his name not be printed, was hit by 585 nm dye laser light that had reflected off an angle-turned frequency doubler when he bent over to adjust a stepper-motor drive. Although his vision has gradually improved, he told *Laser Focus* he lost much of the high-resolution capability in the eye.

The chemist, who's worked with lasers for five years and considers himself a "laser jock," was "amazed" by how little laser energy it took to do so much harm. Measurements made after the accident showed that the pulse back-reflected off the frequency doubler carried only about 25 µJ. But that was enough to punch a hole through multiple layers of eye tissue and to cause hemorrhaging. The result was a blood blister over the macula lutea, the part of the eye that provides visual acuity and that is necessary for tasks such as reading. The pulse energy would have been much higher—close to 2 mJ—if the

NRL group had not earlier taken steps to suppress amplified spontaneous emission in the dye amplifier chain, the victim said.

A surprising—and unsettling—discovery after the accident was how little the doctors knew about laser eye injuries. According to the injured, even retinal specialists were often reduced to guessing during treatment.

The NRL researcher said he never saw a flash when the laser beam struck the eye. "I bent over and all of a sudden I couldn't see," he recalled. *He wasn't wearing safety glasses at the time*, which he said was common practice in the lab. One reason was that the laser—a YAG pumped dye system—was run by computer and seldom needed adjustments which required close eye proximity to the beam. Also, as he pointed out, laser systems that simultaneously produce numerous beams at wavelengths from the ultraviolet to the infrared are difficult to guard against. Since no single pair of goggles will block out all the beams, many lab workers choose to wear none at all. And in a darkened laser room, glasses that protect the wearer from laser light also obscure vision enough to raise the possibility of other hazards, such as hitting your head or tripping over a cable.

The injured chemist criticized laser manufacturers for their method of compliance with Bureau of Radiological Health safety rules. Lasers are built in such a way "that to use one you've usually got to partly disassemble it," he said. "Laser companies should design their product so that it can actually be adjusted and used while complying with BRH rules." He also had harsh words for the maker of the frequency doubler that reflected into his eye. "A $10 beam-stop on that doubler could have prevented this whole thing from happening," he said.

Case History 4 (*Ophthalmology*, February 1981)

On June 27, 1979, a 31-year-old man with five years' experience with lasers sustained a neodymium laser burn to the left eye, causing an immediate dense central scotoma (blind spot).

Circumstances of the injury were as follows: The patient was working on a commercial laser production line adjusting a laser through an opening in its top; this location required him to lean over the laser during beam alignment. In this position his *safety glasses slid up*, allowing the laser beam to pass underneath. The beam was reportedly being reflected from a piece of test paper in a plastic bag, a normal procedure during beam alignment, when the patient heard a snap and saw a bright after image which lasted for 20 minutes before fading into a central scotoma.

The laser was neodymium: YAG with a wavelength of 1.06 μm and a power of 1500 mW. Beam diameter was 500 μm with a pulse duration of 0.1 sec and a rate of about 10 pulses per second.

Case History 5 (*Ophthalmology*, February 1981)

On January 10, 1977, a 32-year-old man with nine years experience with lasers was injured in the left eye by a neodymiumYAG laser causing the immediate onset of photopsias, pain, and visual blur.

Circumstances of the injury were as follows: A laser had been custom designed and built by the patient and others for his company. During modifications, a special beam-turning prism had been added, which incidentally had produced known stray reflections. Plans to block these reflections had not been carried out. The patient, who was *not wearing safety glasses*, had just entered the room to help align the beam when he felt a "pop" and a sudden pain which lasted a few moments and which was associated with many photopsias and floaters.

The laser was Q-switched neodymium:YAG with wavelength of 1.06 μm and peak power of 1 MW (6 mJ per pulse). Pulse duration was 6 ns with 10 pulses per second. Beam diameter was estimated as 1.5 to 3 mm.

Case History 6 (*Ophthalmology*, February 1981)

On December 9, 1979, a 27-year-old graduate student with three years of experience with lasers sustained a neodymium laser burn to his left eye, causing an immediate central scotoma.

Circumstances of the injury were as follows: The patient had assembled an experimental laser and had removed a beam block while making adjustments. As he leaned over, he saw a flash in his peripheral vision and instinctively turned his eye towards the flash. There was an immediate central scotoma and decrease in visual acuity. *He was not wearing safety glasses* at the time of injury.

The laser was pulsed neodymium YAG with a wavelength of

1.06 µm and a power of one mJ with 59 to 100 kW peak power. Beam diameter was 2.5 mm and duration was 20 ns, pulsing at probably 10 pulses per second.

Case History 7 (*Ophthalmology*, February 1981)

On April 15, 1971, a 31-year-old man with many years experience with lasers was struck in the left eye with an argon laser beam, causing an immediate paracentral visual blur.

Circumstances of the injury were as follows: *Without wearing his safety glasses*, the patient was inspecting a clear glass laser beam splitter for dust particles as part of the normal production line procedure. During this examination, laser power was accidentally turned on by another person, causing the beam to strike the patient's eye.

The laser was continuous-wave argon with wavelengths of 488 nm and 514.5 nm. Power incident on the cornea was 70 mW, and beam diameter was 1.4 mm. The exposure duration depended on the blink reflex of the patient, estimated as being 0.125 seconds.

Case History 8 (*Ophthalmology*, February 1981)

On April 21, 1978, a 24-year-old man with five months of experience with lasers was struck in the right eye with an argon laser beam, causing an immediate visual blur and scotoma.

Circumstances of the injury were as follows: The patient was working *without safety glasses* on a laser production line aligning the beam when a reflection from a Brewster window struck his eye, causing him temporarily to see a flash towards which he instinctively looked, bringing on the injury.

The laser was continuous-wave argon with wavelengths of 488 nm and 514.5 nm. Power was 500 mW. Reflection from the Brewster window was estimated to be less than or equal to 25 mW. Beam diameter at the time of injury was probably less than one mm.

Case History 9 (*Ophthalmology*, February 1981)

On August 27, 1979, a 34-year-old man with six years experience with lasers was injured in the left eye with a rhodamine dye laser, causing an immediate visual blur and scotoma. The patient was unaware of any other episodes of laser eye injury.

Circumstances of the injury follow: *While not wearing safety glasses*, the patient was adjusting a laser which had been constructed at his place of employment. While he was attaching a piece of cardboard to the laser to block a known light leak, the beam struck his eye, causing him to see an orange flash followed by an immediate scotoma and blur.

The laser was rhodamine pulsed dye with a wavelength of approximately 592 to 594 nm. Power was 0.2 mJ (20 kW power) with a beam diameter of 6 mm. Beam duration was 10 ns with a rate of 10 pulses per second.

Case History 10 (*Ophthalmology*, February 1981)

On February 13, 1979, a 35-year-old man with 16 years of experience with lasers was struck in the right eye with a beam from a krypton ion laser, resulting in an immediate visual blur and scotoma.

Circumstances of the injury were as follows: The patient was assembling a production line laser, and although *he was not wearing safety glasses*, he had removed a safety screen to align the beam. The beam was focused on a jet of ethylene glycol and dimethyl sulfoxide solution when a bubble in the stream deflected the beam towards the patient's eye, causing the injury.

The laser was continuous-wave krypton ion with a wavelength of 647.1 and 674.2 nm and power of approximately 5 W. The portion of the beam reflected to the patient's eye is unknown. Beam diameter in the fluid was 30 µm.

Summary of Case Histories

The most important factor in each case history is the need for users of lasers to guard vigilantly against potential hazards. In each case history, the user was an experienced laser operator. Even after years of hands-on experience and operation, these users made mistakes that led to damaged eyesight. *You must always assess the potential danger of any experiment that is being performed using lasers.*

Before you turn a laser on, be sure to sign off on the safety checklist. Reduce the beam power whenever necessary and use beam blocks, goggles, and enclosures when possible. Each of the case histories described how the user did not have goggles when operating the laser. Most experienced users often avoid using goggles except when they deem it necessary. But as the case histories show, your eyes will receive the consequences of any mistake that you make.

In some instances you will not be able to see the beam when goggles are worn. If this is the case, be sure to reduce the beam strength to a Class II laser classification for visible lasers, and as low as possible for UV and IR lasers. Place beam blocks wherever stray beams can leave the work area. Be sure to use safety lights to warn visitors or colleagues of laser operation. Never remove beam blocks in the laser cavity to perform needed maintenance unless absolutely necessary. When you do, be sure to use goggles or some other mechanism mentioned above to assure your safety. *Do not take foolish chances. Always think of safety first.*

The case histories illustrate emphatically the need to be alert—always.

Exposure Limits

We now turn our attention to calculating the exposure limit for various lasers and exposure times. These exposure limits will give the amount of energy flux (J/cm^2), or in some cases, the heat flux (W/cm^2) that the eye can handle before a significant probability for damage exists. Several situations must be considered before calculations can be made. Ask the following questions:

1. Does the laser emit light in the visible region?

2. Does the laser emit light as a continuous wave or a train of pulses?

3. Does the pulse repetition frequency (PRF) exceed 1 hertz?

Table 5 (from the American National Standard Institute—ANSI) can be used, along with certain correction factors, to calculate the exposure limits (ELs) for various laser situations once the foregoing questions have been answered. If a need arises to determine the actual energy entering the eye to compare with the EL, assume a worst case situation; that is, use a 7 mm (dark-adapted) pupil. In fact, the ELs found in Table 5 should be converted to power (W) for a pupil size of 7 mm.

Spectral Region	Wavelength	Exposure Time (t), Seconds	Exposure Limits
UV-C	200–280 nm	10^{-9} - 3×10^{4}	3 mJ/cm^2*
UV-B	280–302 nm	10^{-9} - 3×10^{4}	3 mJ/cm^2*
	303 nm	10^{-9} - 3×10^{4}	4 mJ/cm^2*
	304 nm	10^{-9} - 3×10^{4}	6 mJ/cm^2*
	305 nm	10^{-9} - 3×10^{4}	10 mJ/cm^2*
	306 nm	10^{-9} - 3×10^{4}	16 mJ/cm^2*
	307 nm	10^{-9} - 3×10^{4}	25 mJ/cm^2*
	308 nm	10^{-9} - 3×10^{4}	40 mJ/cm^2*
	309 nm	10^{-9} - 3×10^{4}	63 mJ/cm^2*
	310 nm	10^{-9} - 3×10^{4}	100 mJ/cm^2*
	311 nm	10^{-9} - 3×10^{4}	160 mJ/cm^2*
	312 nm	10^{-9} - 3×10^{4}	250 mJ/cm^2*
	313 nm	10^{-9} - 3×10^{4}	400 mJ/cm^2*
	314 nm	10^{-9} - 3×10^{4}	630 mJ/cm^2*
UV-A	315–400 nm	10^{-9} - 3×10^{4}	$0.56 t^{0.25}$ J/cm^2*
	315–400 nm	10^{-9} - 3×10^{4}	1 J/cm^2*
Visible	400–700 nm	10^{-9} - 1.8×10^{-5}	5×10^{-4} mJ/cm^2
	400–700 nm	1.8×10^{-5} - 10	$1.8 t^{0.75}$ mJ/cm^2
	400–550 nm	10 - 10^{4}	10 mJ/cm^2
	550–700 nm	10 - T_1	$1.8 t^{0.75}$ mJ/cm^2
	550–700 nm	T_1 - 10^{4}	$10 C_B$ mJ/cm^2
	400–700 nm	10^{4} - 3×10^{4}	$C_B \times 10^{-3}$ mW/cm^2
IR-A	700–1050 nm	10^{-9} - 1.5×10^{-5}	$5 C_A \times 10^{-4}$ mJ/cm^2
	700–1050 nm	1.8×10^{-5} - 10^{3}	$1.8 C_A t^{0.75}$ mJ/cm^2
	1051–1400 nm	10^{-9} - 5×10^{-5}	5×10^{-3} mJ/cm^2
	1051–1400 nm	5×10^{-5} - 10^{3}	$9 t^{0.75}$ mJ/cm^2
	700–1400 nm	10^{3} - 3×10^{4}	$320 C_A \times 10^{-3}$ W/cm^2
IR-B and C	1.4–1000 mm	10^{-9} - 10^{-7}	10^{-2} J/cm^2
	1.4–1000 mm	10^{-7} - 10	$0.56 t^{0.25}$ J/cm^2
	1.4–1000 mm	>10	0.1 W/cm^2

$C_A = 10^{[0.002(\lambda-700\ nm)]}$ for 700 nm $< \lambda < 1050$ nm, $C_A = 5$ for $1050 < \lambda < 1400$ nm

$C_B = 1$ for $\lambda = 400$ to 500 nm; $C_B = 10^{[0.015(\lambda-550\ nm)]}$ for $\lambda = 550$ to 700 nm

$T_1 = 10$ s for $\lambda = 400$ to 550 nm; $T_1 = 10 \times 10^{[0.02(\lambda-550\ nm)]}$ for $\lambda = 550$ to 700 nm

for $\lambda = 1.5$ to 1.6 µm increase EL by 100, $C_p = n^{-0.25}$, n is the number of pulses

* or $0.56 t^{0.25}$ J/cm^2, whichever is lower.

Table 5.   Exposure Limit (ANSI Z136.1-1993)

The equations in Table 5 can be used for continuous-wave lasers and, with the appropriate corrections, for pulsed lasers. For pulsed lasers, we need the following limitations:

1. The EL for a group of pulses is calculated as a single pulse of the same duration as the entire pulse group. Therefore, add up the total time the pulses are "on" and use the appropriate equation from Table 5. If the radiation is in the visible range, use the blink response time for the total length of exposure time. If the radiation is not in the visible range, then another approximation for the exposure time must be used. Use an exposure time of 10 seconds for infrared lasers. Check the values calculated here with the EL found for just a single pulse in the train. Use the most conservative value, which for most cases will be the single-pulse case.

2. If the frequencies of the pulses, pulse repetition frequency (PRF), exceed 1 Hz, the EL for each pulse is multiplied by a correction factor, C_p. First calculate the number of pulses during the exposure time. For visible lasers, use the blink response time and the PRF. For infrared lasers, use 10 seconds and the PRF. Calculate C_p using the number of pulses, n, where

$$C_p = n^{-0.25}$$

Ultraviolet pulsed lasers have different requirements. The exposure effect on the eye is cumulative over a 24-hour period. ANSI standards [1] require that the EL for a single pulse be reduced by 2.5 in this situation. This assumes that exposures are possible over the next day.

Now consider some examples. The purpose of these examples is to help you learn to perform the calculations necessary to check the safety of any potential eye hazard situation. The examples are also presented to help you better understand the concepts described above. Let's begin by working with some of the case histories listed earlier. First, calculate the EL for the laser in question and then compare the value with the energy flux that actually struck the cornea. Make these calculations yourself. This is the only way to really appreciate the theory and its application. After studying each example, use SAFETY.BAS to compare answers and become familiar with the program.

EXAMPLE 2

Case History 1

This case history shows the damage that can be inflicted on an eye even with a low-energy pulsed laser. The 6 mJ emitted from the laser was a very low level beam; however, it was enough to cause severe damage. Let's calculate the average power and energy flux incident on the eye with this laser and compare them to the safe limits for the eye using this laser. Notice that this laser emits in the IR-A region that is focusable on the retina, but does not invoke a blink response.

Solution

   Laser/wavelength—Nd:YAG/1064 nm, invisible, IR-A

   Pulsed or continuous wave—pulsed, single

   Exposure time—10 ns

   Actual energy or power—6 mJ

   Probable beam diameter—1.5 mm

From Table 5 we notice that a Nd:YAG laser is an IR-A type laser that requires using the following equation,

$$EL = (5 \times 10^{-6}) \ J/cm^2$$

For a 7 mm pupil with an exposure time of 10 ns we get a power of

$$A_p = \pi/4(0.7)^2 \ cm^2 = \text{pupil area}, \ 10^{-8} \ \text{sec exposure time}$$

$$\text{power} = (5 \times 10^{-6} \ J/cm^2) \, A_p \ cm^2/10^{-8} \ \text{sec} = 192 \ W$$

The *actual energy flux* at the cornea that the patient experienced in this case was

$$6 \times 10^{-3} \ J/[\pi(0.15 \ cm)^2/4] = 0.34 \ J/cm^2$$

and the *actual power* over the pulse duration was

$$(0.34 \ J/cm^2)(\pi/4)(0.15 \ cm)^2/10^{-8} = 0.6 \ MW$$

which is several orders of magnitude above the same safe exposure limit! No wonder the patient experienced damage to his eye.

Note: Since there was only one pulse, C_p was not calculated.

Results for Example 2

Actual	**Safe Limit**
power—0.6 MW	192 W
energy flux—0.34 J/cm^2	5×10^{-6} J/cm^2

Compare these values and appreciate the damaging potential of even a low-power laser.

EXAMPLE 3

Case History 6

This case history provides another example of eye damage incurred by a pulsed laser operating at a seemingly low power level. The laser operates in the IR-A wavelength range. Again, the operator was experienced and knew how to operate the laser safely. The eye damage occurred because the operator became careless.

Solution

Let's calculate the actual energy flux and power levels and compare them to the safe operating levels for the eye using this laser. In this example, the correction factor for pulsed lasers is used. This factor reduces the safe operating limit, due to the effects of short time duration pulses that produce shock wave effects in the eye.

Laser/wavelength—Nd:YAG/1064 nm, IR-A
Pulsed or continuous wave—pulsed, 10 per second
Exposure time—20 ns per pulse, PRF = 10
Actual energy or power—1 mJ per pulse
Probable beam diameter—2.5 mm

The most conservative EL will be the one for a single pulse rate with the C_p correction. Using the appropriate equation from Table 5,

$$EL = (5 \times 10^{-6})\, C_p \text{ J/cm}^2$$

The number of pulses can be calculated using PRF = 10 and an exposure time of 10 sec. The 10 sec is used because the laser emits infrared light. This leads to $n = 100$ pulses. $C_p = n^{-0.25} = 0.32$,

$$EL = 1.6 \times 10^{-6} \text{ J/cm}^2$$

which is noticeably less than the actual level seen by the patient. The power for a 7 mm pupil based upon the EL is

$$A_p = [\pi/4(0.7)^2] \text{ cm}^2 = 0.3848 \text{ cm}^2 = \text{pupil area}$$

$$A_b = [\pi/4(0.25)^2] \text{ cm}^2 = 0.0491 \text{ cm}^2 = \text{beam area}$$

$$\text{power} = (1.6 \times 10^{-6} \text{ J/cm}^2)A_p \text{ cm}^2/(2 \times 10^{-8} \text{ sec}) = 30 \text{ W}$$

The *actual power* seen for 1 pulse was

$$(1 \times 10^{-3} \text{ J})/(2 \times 10^{-8} \text{ sec}) = 50 \text{ kW}$$

The *actual energy flux* seen for 1 pulse was

$$1 \text{ mJ}/[(0.25 \text{ cm})^2 (\pi/4)] = 20.4 \text{ mJ/cm}^2$$

Results for Example 3

Actual	**Safe Limit**
power—50 kW	30 W (0.03 kW), pulsed
energy flux—0.0204 J/cm^2	1.6 x 10^{-6} J/cm^2

EXAMPLE 4

Case History 8

This example shows the damage produced by the reflection of a laser, off a Brewster window, at a power level of only 25 mW. Consider the power output of a light bulb. Operating at 50 W, the light bulb would appear to provide a much greater danger than the reflection from a laser providing only 25 mW. Remember that a light bulb is an extended source. Example 1 showed the difference between a collimated source, such as a laser, and an extended source, such as a light bulb. Let's calculate the acceptable safe eye limits for this laser and then compare them to the actual power and energy flux levels.

Solution

> Laser/wavelength—Ar/488 nm, visible
> Pulsed or continuous wave—continuous
> Exposure time—0.25 seconds, blink response
> Actual energy or power—25 mW
> Probable beam diameter—1 mm

From Table 5 the exposure limit for a diffraction limited eye is

$$\text{EL} = 1.8(t^{3/4}) \text{ mJ/cm}^2 = 0.64 \text{ mJ/cm}^2$$

using a blink response of 0.25 sec while the *actual exposure* for this case history was

$$(25 \text{ mW})(0.25 \text{ sec})/[\pi/4(0.1 \text{ cm})^2] = 796 \text{ mJ/cm}^2$$

which is well above the safe level set by the exposure limit. The corresponding safe power limit for a 7 mm pupil is calculated as

$$A_p = [(\pi/4)(0.7)]^2 \text{ cm}^2 = 0.3848 \text{ cm}^2$$

$$\text{power} = (0.64 \times 10^{-3} \text{ mJ/cm}^2)A_p /0.25 \text{ sec} = 1 \text{ mW}$$

while the power for the actual case was 25 mW. *Notice* from the calculation for the continuous-wave laser that the EL leads to an upper safe power limit for the eye of 1 mW, which is the Class II/III dividing line. This was no accident. The safe power limits were calculated from the exposure limits.

Results for Example 4

Actual	**Safe Limit**
power—25 mW	1 mW
energy flux—795 mJ/cm^2	0.64 mJ/cm^2

Further examples can be found in Safety with *Lasers and Other Optical Sources* by Sliney and Wolbarsht [15]. The *Laser Safety Guide* [9], published by the Laser Institute of America, is another useful reference. The computer programs in Appendix B should also be useful for safety-related questions.

REFERENCES

1. American National Standard Institute. *Safe Use of Lasers*, ANSI Z136.1-1993. New York: ANSI, 1993.

2. Graymore, Clive. *Biochemistry of the Eye*. New York: Academic Press, 1970.

3. Hecht, Eugene. *Optics*, 2nd ed. Reading, MA: Addison-Wesley, 1987.

4. Incropera, Frank, and David DeWitt. *Fundamentals of Heat and Mass Transfer*, 3rd ed. New York: John Wiley, 1989.

5. Jenkins, Francis, and Harvey White. *Fundamentals of Optics*, 4th ed. New York: McGraw-Hill, 1976.

6. Lappin, P. W. "Ocular Damage Thresholds for the Helium–Neon Laser." *Archives of Environmental Health*, Vol. 20 (February 1970), pp. 177–183.

7. Lappin, P. W., and P. S. Coogan. *Archives of Ophthalmology*, Vol. 84 (September 1970), pp. 350–354.

8. *Laser Focus World* (*Laser Focus* before 1989). Published PennWell Publishing Company, 1421 S. Sheridan, Tulsa, Oklahoma 74112.

9. Laser Institute of America. *Laser Safety Guide*, fifth printing, January 1992. Available from the Institute, 12424 Research Parkway, Suite 130, Orlando, Florida 32826.

10. Mihran, R. T. "Interaction of Laser Radiation with Structures of the Eye." *IEEE Transactions on Education*, Vol. 34, no. 3 (August 1991), pp. 250–259.

11. National Institute of Standards and Technology. *Self-study Manual on Optical Radiation Measurements.* National Bureau of Standards Technical Note 910-2, Part 1, Concepts, Chapters 4 and 5, February 1978.

12. National Society for the Prevention of Blindness. *Teaching About Blindness.* New York: The Society, 1972.

13. *Opthalmology* (published by the American Academy of Ophthalmology). "Retinal Injury due to Industrial Laser Burns," authored by Edwin Boldrey, Hunter Little, Milton Flocks, and Arthur Vassiliadis, Vol. 88 (1981), pp. 101–107.

14. Siegel, Robert, and John Howell. *Thermal Radiation Heat Transfer,* 3rd ed. Bristol, PA: Hemisphere, 1992.

15. Sliney, David, and Myron Wolbarsht. *Safety with Lasers and Other Optical Sources, A Comprehensive Handbook.* New York: Plenum Press, 1981.

16. Winburn, D. C. *Practical Laser Safety.* New York: Marcel Dekker, 1985.

17. Verdeyen, J. T. *Laser Electronics.* Englewood Cliffs, NJ: Prentice Hall, 1981.

18. Yariv, Amnon. *Optical Electronics,* 3rd ed. New York: Holt, Rinehart and Winston, 1985.

SAFETY PROCEDURES

Appoint a safety officer for the lab (well trained).

Post lab safety rules for all to see.

Label all lasers with classification and wavelength information.

Wear eye protection (provide glasses at each laser station).

Enclose beam path (beam blocks).

Reduce beam power level using ND filters during alignment.

Hazard signs (see examples) and lights

Door interlocks

Place the beam paths at levels below or above the natural standing or sitting positions to avoid inadvertent exposures.

Restrict area access.

Permit no fooling around.

Permit no liquids or food in the lab area.

Post the emergency phone numbers and procedures for handling safety problems.

Require all personnel to take safety course and pass a written and oral exam.

Safety Signs and Labels

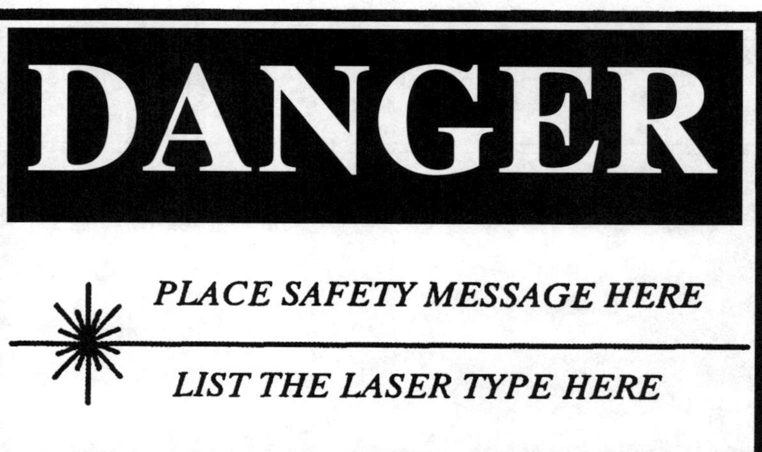

Use the preceding sign for Class III and Class IV lasers.

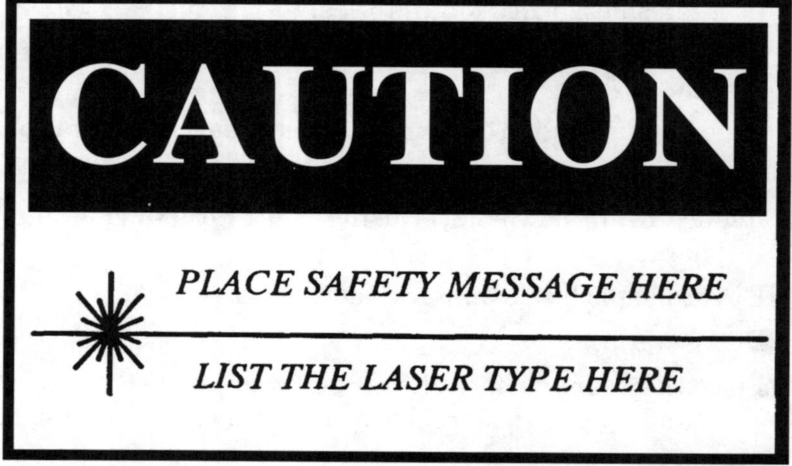

Use the preceding sign for lower-power lasers.

The high-power laser signs should use red colors to emphasize the danger associated with their use. The lower-power laser should use yellow to match the caution emphasis. These signs can be ordered from the Laser Institute of America. See the References section for the address.

QUESTIONS ON LASER & EYE SAFETY

Aspects of the Eye

1. Describe convection heat transfer and the role it plays in regulating the temperature of the eye. Write the basic equation that describes convection heat transfer and describe each term. If the retina is heated up by a laser to 40 °C, what will be the necessary heat transfer, in watts, that the blood flow must carry off to return the retina to its initial temperature? Assume that blood flow with a temperature of 37 °C and a convection heat transfer coefficient in the blood vessel of 25 W/m²-C. Also assume that the surface area over which the heat is transferred is equal to 0.0004 m².

2. Make a sketch of the human eye and label several (at least 15) of its components. What is the concentration ratio of the cornea and lens for collimated light? Since the Sun is an extended source, it does not emit collimated light. Light from the Sun can be considered to be contained in a cone of angle 0.0092 radians (approximately 0.5 degrees). Given this cone angle and knowing the effective focal length of the eye, calculate the size of the Sun's image on the retina. What is the size of the image of a 1 mm laser beam? Explain the difference between light leaving an extended source and a collimated beam of light. A sketch might help. Calculate the energy flux on the retina from the concentrated sunlight. Compare this to the safe operating limit for a visible, continuous-wave laser. Assume a blink response of 0.25 sec and a daylight-size pupil. Also assume that the flux coming from the Sun and striking the cornea is 1 kW/m².

3. "Different structures of the eye may be injured depending upon which structure absorbs the greatest radiant energy per volume of tissue." Given this statement, which parts of the eye absorb most of the energy from a Nd:YAG laser and which part will be damaged the most? What is the wavelength from such a laser?

4. What components of the eye are the most susceptible to the ultraviolet (UV-A, UV-B, UV-C) or far-infrared (IR-B, IR-C) portions of the electromagnetic spectrum? Why does IR-A radiation pose such a problem for eye safety?

5. What are the four classes of laser classification? Give a brief description of each. What is the blink reflex time of the eye?

6. Under what classification would you place a helium–neon laser with a power level of 0.5 mW? What classification would you use for 15 and 50 mW helium–neon lasers? How would you classify a 4 W argon laser? How about a 2 mJ Nd:YAG laser?

7. Which part of the eye performs most of the refraction of the incoming visible radiation? What percentage of the total refraction is performed by this part of the eye? What is the refractive power of the relaxed normal eye? Define diopter.

8. If the cornea is slightly damaged by dust or some other device, is it capable of repairing itself? How long does this process take? Sketch the cornea and label its parts. Also show which part is capable of regeneration.

9. The aqueous humor acts as a filter and heat exchanger for the eye. Explain how glaucoma can be caused by the aqueous humor, in particular describe the function of the trabecular meshwork and the canal of Schlemm.

10. The lens is not a solid crystalline object, but is composed of layers much like an onion. What is accommodation? How is accommodation lost (by a natural process)? If the lens contracts a cataract it is often replaced with an artificial solid lens. This is normally an operation performed on older people. Obviously, accommodation is lost, but is this really of much concern for older people? Why?

11. What happens to the gel-like vitreous humor if it comes in contact with blood? What can cause the vitreous to contract?

12. What are the two types of retinal photoreceptor cells? How many of each are there, and what are their sizes? What part of the eye do you use when reading? Where is the highest concentration of cones? What functions do they perform? What good are the attributes of rods? Which part of the eye is the "garbage collector"? What do we mean by garbage collector?

13. How does a detached retina occur? Between which components of the eye does this detachment take place?

14. Which component of the eye provides the temperature stabilization through blood flow (main heat exchanger)? What is scotoma? How are scotomas generated?

15. What is the name of the white portion of the eye? Which part of the eye acts as the aperture stop?

16. What is the pupil size for the normal dark-adapted eye? What is the pupil size for the normal daylight-adapted eye? What is the shortest time that the iris can contract when exposed to a bright light source?

17. What is the power limit between Class III and Class IV lasers? Power output at or greater than this level is capable of damaging skin, even over short (1 sec) time periods. Notice that this level is not as high as you might think. What is the power output of a standard incandescent light bulb?

18. From Case Histories 4, 5, 7, 9, and 10 calculate the EL and the equivalent power for each type of laser. Then compare the results with the actual power received by the patient. Note the difference.

Experimental Procedure

1. What are the safety regulations for your lab?

2. Name at least 12 of the major components of the lab. Include the manufacturer and a brief description of each component.

3. A 50 mW helium–neon laser has the following specifications:
    a. Output power—50 mW
    b. Wavelength—0.633 μm
    c. Beam diameter—2 mm @ $1/e^2$
    d. Polarization—linear to 1 part in 10, oriented vertically

    Calculate the total energy/area that can be absorbed by the retina over a period of time corresponding to the blink response of the eye. How does this compare to the EL for this laser? How fast would the eye have to respond to be safe? How low a power level would you have to take the laser (by using Nd filters) to be safe?

4. A 15 mW helium–neon laser has the following specifications:
    a. Output power—15 mW
    b. Wavelength—0.633 μm
    c. Beam diameter—1.2 mm @ $1/e^2$
    d. Polarization—linear to 1 part in 10, oriented vertically to 5 degrees.

    Perform the same calculations as in part 3.

Accommodation (ah-kom'o-da' shun). Adjustment of the eye for seeing objects at various distances, accomplished by altering the shape of the crystalline lens by action of the ciliary muscle, thus changing its power and focusing a clear image on the retina.

Amblyopia (am'ble-o'pe-ah). Diminished vision without a detectable lesion or disease of the eye.

Amblyopia ex Anopsia (ex-anop'sia). Amblyopia acquired through lack of use of the eye.

Anterior Chamber (an-tir'e-r). Space in the front of the eye, bounded in front by the cornea and behind by the iris, filled with aqueous.

Anterior Segment. Includes the cornea, conjunctiva, aqueous humor, iris and lens.

Aqueous humor (a'kwe-us). The clear, watery fluid filling the anterior and posterior chambers of the anterior segment of the eye. It helps cleanse the lens and cornea. It also serves as a heat-absorbing water filter for the lens.

Astigmatism (ah-stig'mah-tizm). Faulty vision caused by imperfections in the curvature of the cornea that prevent light rays from focusing at a single point on the retina; instead they are focused separately. If rays focus in front of the retina, this is called myopia and if rays focus behind the retina, this is called hyperopia. In lenses, astigmatism is a third-order monochromatic aberration.

Blepharitis (blef'ah-ri'tis). Inflammation of the eyelids.

Blind spot. See optic disk, scotoma.

Cataract (kat'ah-rakt). Loss of transparency of the lens of the eye or its capsule, resulting in partial or total blindness.

> *incipient cataract* early stages of formation, or regions of opaque sectors surrounded by clear spaces.
> *congenital cataract* developed before birth.
> *senile cataract* lens hardens as we get older and it becomes opaque.

Choroid (kor'oyd). The vascular, intermediate coat that furnishes nourishment to the other parts of the eyeball. The primary function of the blood in the choroid is to keep the eye warm and at a uniform temperature.

Ciliary Body (sil'-e-er-e). Portion of the vascular coat between the iris and the choroid. It consists of ciliary processes and the ciliary muscle. Aqueous is replenished largely by secretion from the ciliary body.

Cones and Rods. The two types of light-sensitive nerve endings that are present in the retina and make it possible for it to transmit visual impulses to the brain. Cones are sensitive to fine detail and color; rods are concerned with motion and vision at low degrees of illumination (as in night vision). There are approximately 6,000,000 cones and 125,000,000 rods in the entire retina.

Congenital (kon-jen'i-tal). Present at birth.

Conjunctiva (kon-junk'ti-vah). The thin transparent mucous membrane lining the inner surface of the eyelids (palpebral conjunctiva) and the exposed surface of the anterior sclera up to the border of the cornea (bulbar conjunctiva); the epithelial layer of the conjunctiva is continuous with the corneal epithelium.

Conjunctival discharge (of the eye). The eyeball experiences an increased secretion of mucus from its surface.

Conjunctivitis (kon-junk-ta'vit-es). Inflammation of the conjunctiva resulting from bacterial, viral, or allergic agents; for example, acute catarrhal conjunctivitis is caused by a bacterium (usually pneumococcus).

Cornea (kor'ne-ah). The transparent anterior part of the outer coat of the eyeball that serves as the major refracting medium; it contains five layers (epithelium, Bowmen's membrane, stroma, Descemet's membrane, and corneal endothelium); corneas donated for transplantation are now routinely preserved at eye banks.

Corneal graft. Operation to restore vision by replacing a section of opaque cornea with transparent cornea.

Diopter (D) (di-op'ter). The reciprocal of the effective focal length expressed in meters; used to designate the refractive power of a lens or an optical system.

Diplopia (dy-plo'pe-ah). Double vision; that is, perception of two images of a single object.

Dyslexia (dis-lek'se-ah). Inability to read or group the meaning of written or printed words.

Edema (i-de'm-ah). Excessive fluid in body cavities or tissues.

Emmetropia (em-e-tro'pe-ah). The normal condition of the refractive system of the eye in which the light rays entering the eyeball focus exactly on the retina.

Endothelium (en'do-the'le-um). A thin layer of cells lining various cavities, blood vessels, and lymph vessels.

Enucleation (e-nu'kle-a'shun). The surgical removal of a tumor or of an organ, such as the eyeball, in its entirety, without rupture.

Epithelium (ep'i-the'le-um). The nonvascular cellular layer that covers the internal and external surfaces of the body.

Erythema (er'i-the'mah). Redness of the skin.

Esotropia (es-o-tro'pe-ah). Convergent strabismus; strabismus in which the eye deviates inward, toward the nose.

Etiology (e'te-ol'o-je). The study of causes, specifically the cause of a disease.

Exposure. Irradiance times time $(Ir * t)$, with units of energy/area or J/cm^2. The exposure relates the energy arriving from the light source to the area being irradiated.

Exposure Limit. The limit at which the eye can safely survive irradiation from a light source.

Exophthalmos (ek'sof-thal'mus). Abnormal protrusion of the eyeballs from their sockets.

Exotropia (ek-so-tro'pe-ah). Divergent strabismus; strabismus in which the eye deviates outward.

Fluence. The flow of radiant energy across a projected area, as opposed to the actual area. Fluence is a quantity that is part of the radiometric system of units. It is the intensity integrated over direction and time. The units are joules per meter squared.

Fovea centralis (fo've-ah). An area approximately 1.5 mm in diameter in the macula lutea of the retina; it is the area of greatest visual acuity. This is where the highest concentration of cone receptors exist and are responsible for not only color but also vision of greatest acuity.

Fundus (fun'dus). The interior surface of the eye (or any organ), in this case the retina.

Glaucoma (glaw-ko'mah). A group of eye diseases characterized by an increase in intraocular pressure, due to restricted outflow of the aqueous humor through the trabecular meshwork and spaces of Fontana in the anterior chamber angle (between the root of the iris and cornea).

Heterophoria (het'er-o-fo're-ah). The tendency of the optic axis to deviate toward or away from each other.

Heterotropia (het-e-ro'tro-pee-ah). A visual disorder in which one eye cannot focus with the other. Also called strabismus.

Hydrophthalmos (hi' dro-fth). A condition marked by an increase of intraocular fluid with enlargement of the eyeball and protrusion of the cornea. Also called congenital glaucoma.

Hyperopia (hi'per-o'pe-ah). A condition of the eye in which parallel light rays entering the eyeball focus behind the retina, because the eyeball is short or the refractive power of the lens is weak. Also called hypermetropia; farsightedness.

Iris (i'ris). The doughnut-shaped part of the eye, situated between the cornea and crystalline lens, and separating the anterior and posterior chambers; the contraction of the iris alters the size of the pupil; the amount of pigment in it determines the color of the eye.

Iritis (i-ri'tis). Inflammation of the iris; condition marked by pain.

Keratitis (ker'ah-ti'tis). Inflammation of the cornea. Also called corneitis, often characterized by dullness and the loss of transparency.

Lacrimal gland (lak'ri-mal). A gland that secretes tears; located in the upper lateral portion of the orbit.

Lacrimation (lak'ri-ma'shun). The secretion, especially excessive, of tears.

Lenticular (len-tik'u-lar). Relating to a lens.

Lesion (le'zhun). An abnormal structural change in the body due to injury or disease.

Macula lutea (mak'u-lah). A small oval yellowish depression on the retina, lateral to and slightly below the optic disk; it contains the fovea centralis. Also called macula retinae, yellow spot.

Microphthalmia (mi-krof-thal'me-ah). Abnormal smallness of the eyeballs.

Miosis (mi-o'sis). Reduction in size of the pupil of the eye.

Myopia (mi-o'pe-ah). A condition of the eye in which light rays entering the eyeball from a distance focus in front of the retina, causing only near objects to be seen in focus. Also called nearsight, near-sightedness, shortsightedness.

Nystagmus (nis-tag'mus). An involuntary movement of the eyes in a rotatory, vertical, or horizontal direction.

Ocular fundus. The posterior portion of the interior of the eye.

Optic atrophy (op'tik-at'ro-fe). Wasting away of the optic nerve fibers characterized by pallor of the optic nerve head and accompanied by visual loss.

Optic disk. The pinkish-white oval or circular area of the retina, which is the site of entrance of the optic nerve. Also called blind spot.

Optic nerve. The special nerve of the sense of sight that carries messages from the retina to the brain.

Ophthalmologist (of'thal-mol'o-jist). A physician who specializes in treating diseases and refractive errors of the eye.

Orbit. The cavity in the skull that houses the eyeball.

Photokeratitis. Damage to the outer corneal layer due to short ultraviolet radiation, as occurs in photophthamia (welder's flash).

Photophobia. Abnormal intolerance or fear of light.

Phoria (fo're-ah). A latent tendency toward crossed eyes. Condition not usually observed. See heterophoria.

Photometric units. Are usually associated with the visible and near-visible part of the spectrum. These units tend to be biased to the spectral response of an average observer (typically a younger observer). Photometric measurements are weighted by the spectral response of this average observer.

Photopic (fo-top'ick). Daylight vision with eyes adapted to normal bright light.

Pinguecula (ping-gwek'u-lah). A small, slightly raised, yellowish, nonfatty thickening of the conjunctiva of the eye near the sclerocorneal junction, usually on the nasal side. Most commonly seen in older people.

Posterior chamber. Space between the back of the iris and the front of the lens; filled with aqueous humor.

Posterior segment. Includes the parts of the eye behind the lens (vitreous, fovea, sclera, choroid, retina, macula, optic disk, optic nerve and retinal pigment epithelium).

Presbyopia (pres'be-o'pe-ah). Diminution of accommodation power in the eyes due to advancing age.

Pterygium (te-rij'e-um). A horizontal, triangular growth of the bulbar conjunctiva; a slowly advancing lesion, believed to be caused by ultraviolet radiation.

Ptosis (to'sis). A drooping of the upper lid due to weakness or paralysis of a portion (or branch) of the third nerve that controls the levator muscle that raises the lid.

Pupil (pew'pil). The circular opening in the center of the iris, through which light enters the eye. The pupil acts as an aperture stop ranging in size from 2 mm to 8 mm.

Radiant exitance. The radiant power leaving the surface. The surface emits power based upon its temperature. The units are watts per meter squared. The power emitted per meter squared is referred to as radiant exitance, whereas the power incident on a surface per meter squared is referred to as irradiance. The difference being mainly whether the radiation was emitted or incident on the surface.

Radiant intensity. In radiometric units, defined as the power flowing through a solid angle. This is the intensity integrated over the projected area. The units are watts per steradian.

Radiometric units. These units deal with the general radiant energy spectral regime. These units are widely used among divergent disciplines (physics and engineering). The radiometric system of units are often referred to as the CIE (international agency that sets units, instrument calibration standards, and other related areas) system.

Retina (ret'i-nah). The light-receptive layer and terminal expansion of the optic nerve in the eye. It extends from the point of exit of the nerve forward to the ora serrata.

Retinal detachment (ret'i-nal). The separation of the retina from the underlying vascular or choroid layer of the eye breaking connections between the rods and cones and the pigment layer. Most often the result of a hole or tear in the retina.

Retinal pigment epithelium (RPE). One of the very complex layers of nerve cells that make up the retina; plays a critical role in the retinal metabolism and photochemistry; RPE cells also consume the discs shed by the rods outer segments.

Retinitis (ret'i-ni'tis). Inflammation of the retina.

Retinitis pigmentosa (pig-men-to'sah). Hereditary degeneration and atrophy of the retina, usually with migration of pigment, causing gradual reduction of vision that maybe complete.

Schlemm's canal. A ringlike canal in the anterior edge of the sclera, encircling the cornea; it serves as a drain of excess aqueous humor of the anterior chamber of the eye. Also called the scleral venous sinus.

Sclera (skle'rah). The tough, white membranous tunic that covers all the eyeball except the anterior portion, which is occupied by the cornea.

Scotoma (sko-to'mah). An abnormal blind spot; an area in the visual field in which vision is absent or greatly diminished.

Scotopic (sko-top'ik). Denoting the low levels of illumination to which the eye's sensitivity to light became greatly increased when it is dark adapted. Relating to vision that is adapted to low levels of illumination.

Solid angle. Represents a direction and "slice" of space through which energy can flow. The solid angle can also be thought of as a cone in space, or as a 3-D measure of angle. The steradian is the unit for solid angle.

Squamous (skwa'mus). Scaly; covered with scales; resembling scales.

Stereopsis (ster'e-op'sis). Visual depth perception produced by slight disparateness of images, that is, when images fall on slightly disparate points of the retina.

Strabismus (strah-biz'mus). A visual disorder in which one eye cannot focus with the other. Also called heterotropia.

Stroma (stro'muh). The framework of an organ, usually composed of connective tissue, that supports the functional elements or cells.

Stromal Haze. A condition where the main body of the cornea or the conjunctive tissue becomes clouded.

Suspensory ligaments (sus-pen-so're lig'ah-ments). Ligaments that aid in keeping an organ or part in place.

Trabecular meshwork (trah-bek'u-lar). Patch of loose network made up of the iris connective tissue, fibers of the sclera, and fine fibers of Descemet's membrane lined by endothelial cells. This meshwork constitutes the main exit route for aqueous humor from the anterior chamber, which passes through it to reach the canal of Schlemm.

Trachoma (trah-ko'mah). A contagious infection of the conjunctiva and cornea, producing loss of vision, caused by Chlamydia trachomatis (bacteria).

Appendix B — Computer Programs

Several examples are worked in this appendix. They are used primarily to demonstrate the use of the computer programs that can be used with this book; available on disk from the authors. The reader should work these examples even if the programs are not used. The experience is useful for understanding the material in greater detail. The best procedure is to work the examples first and then refer to the solutions.

The computer programs written to accompany this book are educational in focus. Program TEACH.BAS has a tutorial section for those readers that need reinforcement in geometrical optics. It also has a lens calculation program that uses matrix techniques to determine basic lens parameters and image properties. Program SAFETY.BAS has a section devoted to laser classification and the determination of exposure limits. The next section of the program estimates the heat flux on the retina for different types of sources. These sources include lasers and diffusely emitting objects.

Each program was written in BASIC. BASIC was chosen because most users have it on their computers. BASIC was also chosen because it is a very simple language and any user can learn how to modify these programs easily. The programs are not written efficiently. They are written such that a user can easily change or update any section of the program. We encourage each user to get to know the programs and modify them to meet their needs. We will work example problems that show some of the features of each program. We also suggest that you use the programs to verify the calculations shown in the example problems in the main text of this book.

SAFETY.BAS

Let's begin with program SAFETY.BAS. The program listing is in Appendix C. Choose a laser that is commonly used in the laboratory. A helium–neon laser is a good choice.

> **SAFETY.BAS is not a certified safety program and should be used with care.**

Every lab, no mater how sophisticated or basic, has such a laser. The potential safety hazard to the eye of a helium–neon laser depends on several criteria. The power levels achieved by the helium–neon laser are never high enough to present a danger to the skin. However, the danger to the eye can be very real. Helium–neon lasers can be Class I, Class II, or Class III in classification. Program SAFETY.BAS can help you determine which class the laser is and what hazards it can present to the eye.

Lines 350–480 in the program make an important statement about the program: It is not a certified laser safety program. No guarantees can be made about its accuracy or completeness. It is for educational uses and to help check the levels of various lasers. The program has been checked for many cases and different types of lasers. No errors have been found; however, some may exist. One potential problem area is in the Class I estimates. Not every ANSI feature was added to the program. This was not deemed critical because we have concentrated on the laser classifications that present a danger to the eye. In each case, the program takes a conservative approach to the Class I classification. Therefore, if an error exists, it should be on the safe side.

The program first asks if the eye safety section or the eye model section is to be used. The eye safety section determines the classification of the laser, the exposure limit, the energy flux in the collimated beam, and the limiting aperture. Lines 1400–1900 contain the code for determining the classification for a pulsed laser. Lines 2530–3040 contain the code for continuous-wave lasers. These sections can be easily checked for ultraviolet, visible, and near- and far-infrared wavelength ranges. The classification criteria listed in the code follows ANSI Z136.1-1993. New updates to the standard can be easily incorporated into the code between lines 1400–1900 for pulsed laser and lines 2530–3040 for continuous-wave lasers.

The program asks for the type of laser (pulsed or continuous wave), the pulse repetition rate (PRF, if required), the energy per pulse (if required), the diameter of the laser beam, and the power of the laser (if required). Lines 1340 and 2470 find the energy flux for pulsed and continuous lasers, respectively, from this information.

The exposure limits are found for both pulsed and continuous-wave lasers in the subroutine beginning on line 3520 in the program. The exposure limits are based on wavelength and exposure times. Program SAFETY.BAS uses the blink response time for continuous-wave Class II lasers, 10 seconds for continuous-wave nonvisible lasers, and the pulse duration for pulsed lasers. Ten seconds is the suggested exposure time given by the ANSI standard for nonvisible lasers.

ANSI exposure limits for ultraviolet lasers have wide exposure time limits. Lines 3560–3990 provide the exposure limits for UV lasers. The exposure times are not used by the program for UV lasers because the pulse duration of most lasers used in the lab fall within the listed range. For continuous-wave lasers the 10 second recommendation given by ANSI is also well within the listed range. For these reasons, you will not find exposure times affecting the exposure limit calculations in the program for ultraviolet lasers.

The ANSI standards for visible and infrared lasers include exposure times. The blink response, pulse duration, and 10 second limit are all used by the program in the appropriate areas. Cases where you may want to consider forced, long duration viewing of the laser beam cannot be covered by this program. Forced viewing of the laser must be avoided at all times.

The second part of the program begins at line 4420. This is the simplified model for the eye. The eye is modeled as a thin lens with a focal length of 17 mm. The image size calculations on the retina are found by using the thin lens equation (see [3 and 5] and program TEACH.BAS) and the diffraction limit for perfect lenses. Under no circumstances is the image size allowed to be smaller than the diffraction limit for the perfect eye. The diffraction limit is found in line 5330 in the code.

The program calculates the fluxes for collimated sources such as lasers and for extended sources such as the Sun. The flux values are found on the cornea and the retina. The ratio of the two are calculated to provide the concentration ratio as a measure of the potential danger from any given source. The retinal flux and the corneal flux are calculated on lines 5440 and 5460, respectively.

Let's work some examples now using the program SAFETY.BAS.

EXAMPLE B.1

Laser	**Helium–neon**
Wavelength	0.6328 µm
Power level	50 mW
Pulse duration	Continuous
Beam diameter	2 mm

The foregoing data are used in each part of the program. The first section will determine the class of laser and the exposure limit. The results from the program are

Class	**III**
Energy flux	0.4 J/cm^2
Exposure limit	0.00064 J/cm^2
Power flux	1.6 W/cm^2

The second section of the program determines the spot size on the retina, the heat flux on the retina, the heat flux on the cornea, and the relative concentration. The results from the program are

Retinal spot size	0.0013 cm
Retinal heat flux	3.7 x 10^4 W/cm^2
Corneal heat flux	1.6 W/cm^2
Concentration ratio	23,223

Note that the exposure limit is orders of magnitude lower than the actual energy flux. The laser is a Class III device and a definite eye hazard problem. The spot size on the retina is much smaller than the size of the fovea and capable of burning the photoreceptors attached to it. Note that a heat flux of approximately 2 W/cm^2 is capable of burning paper. *Be careful of this laser. Follow all safety precautions.*

EXAMPLE B.2

Laser	Argon ion
Wavelength	0.514 µm
Power level	2 W
Pulse duration	Continuous
Beam diameter	2 mm

This is a common laser for laboratory applications. It is a continuous-wave laser used for holography, electrooptics, and many other applications. As we will see, this laser must be respected. The results for this case are

Class	IV
Energy flux	15.9 J/cm^2
Exposure limit	0.00064 J/cm^2
Power flux	63.7 W/cm^2

From the second section of the program we get

Retinal spot size	0.0011 cm
Retinal heat flux	2.2 x 10^6 W/cm^2
Corneal heat flux	63.7 W/cm^2
Concentration ratio	35,198

This example shows the extreme difference between the actual energy flux and the exposure limit. The heat flux on the retina is enormous and clearly a hazard to the eye. This is a Class IV laser and also dangerous to the skin. *Treat this laser with respect. Take all necessary safety precautions.*

EXAMPLE B.3

This is an example of a pulsed laser. The Nd:YAG laser is commonly used for a number of applications. In this example the output beam has been frequency doubled to provide a visible wavelength.

Laser	**Nd:YAG**
Wavelength	0.532 µm
Power level	30 MW
Pulse duration	10 ns
Beam diameter	3 mm
Energy pulse	0.3 J
Pulse repetition rate	30 Hz

This laser is capable of producing extremely high fluxes. The power level was determined taking the known energy level per pulse and dividing by the pulse duration. The results from the program are

Class	**IV**
Energy flux	4.2 J/cm^2
Exposure limit	0.0000003 J/cm^2

The energy flux is orders of magnitude higher than the exposure limit. It is clearly a Class IV laser. The results from the second section of the program are

Retinal spot size	0.00095 cm
Retinal heat flux	4.2 x 10^{13} W/cm^2
Corneal heat flux	4.2 x 10^8 W/cm^2
Concentration ratio	100,000

Again, we see that this laser is capable of producing very high heat flux levels. *Remember that Class IV lasers are capable of damaging the eye even with diffuse reflections. Respect this laser.*

Use beam blocks and enclose the laser beam whenever possible. Reduce the power (or energy) of the laser during alignment of the optical system. Be sure that all personnel are aware of the operation of the laser and using the appropriate eye protection. Also, be sure to post warning signs and control access to the testing area.

EXAMPLE B.4

This is essentially the same laser as in the last example. The difference is the output wavelength is 1.064 µm. The is primary wavelength for this laser. As a consequence, the energy per pulse is higher than for the frequency doubled laser in Example B.3.

Laser	**Nd:YAG**
Wavelength	1.064 µm
Power level	100 MW
Pulse duration	10 ns
Beam diameter	3 mm
Energy pulse	1 J
Pulse repetition rate	30 Hz

From this information the program provides the following results

Class	**IV**
Energy flux	14.1 J/cm^2
Exposure limit	0.0000012 J/cm^2

These values are correspondingly higher than for Example B.3. One important difference is the wavelength. This laser is an IR-A device. Even reflections cannot cause the eye to blink due to photon interaction. This is a Class IV laser, which is a clear danger to the eye. The second section of the program provides the following results

Retinal spot size	0.0015 cm
Retinal heat flux	5.9 x 10^{13} W/cm^2
Corneal heat flux	1.4 x 10^9 W/cm^2
Concentration ratio	41,584

Again, *show this laser the respect it deserves!*

EXAMPLE B.5

We will now look at a powerful continuous-wave laser that operates well into the infrared part of the spectrum. It is a CO_2 laser operating at 10.64 µm. The specifications for this laser are

Laser	**Carbon dioxide**
Wavelength	10.64 µm
Power level	500 W
Pulse duration	Continuous
Beam diameter	15 mm

This laser is not as common in the laboratory as the other lasers we have considered. It is used for a variety of applications and is a workhorse in industry. The power level is high for a continuous-wave laser, and the beam diameter is much larger than the other lasers we have considered.

Class	**IV**
Energy flux	2829 J/cm^2
Exposure limit	0.001 J/cm^2
Power flux	283 W/cm^2

This laser is clearly a Class IV device with an extremely high energy flux level. The actual level is several orders of magnitude greater than the exposure limit. Since this laser emits invisible radiation, special care must be taken around work areas to protect from diffuse reflections. A continuous-wave laser, such as this one, can cause a long duration eye hazard problem that can be over looked. *Be careful.*

The next section of the program provides the following results:

Retinal spot size	0.0047 cm
Retinal heat flux	2.8 x 10^7 W/cm^2
Corneal heat flux	282.9 W/cm^2
Concentration ratio	100,000

A carbon dioxide laser is a very dependable device with a reputation of operating for years without problems. But along with the dependability of the laser, the safety problems are often ignored or overlooked. *Remember the lessons from the case histories. Do not take laser safety for granted.*

EXAMPLE B.6

We will now consider sources that are not lasers. These sources are considered to be diffuse reflectors and are called extended sources. The images on the retina are larger in size than those provided by collimated sources. The average heat and energy fluxes are correspondingly lower since the same amount of power and energy are distributed over a greater area.

In this example the Sun is the source. The power level was calculated for a 7 mm pupil and a solar flux of 1000 W/m^2. This solar flux is a common value around noon time.

Source	Sun
Wavelength	Visible
Power level (cornea)	0.039 W
Distance to object	149,025,249,631 m
Diameter of object	1,391,168,408 m

The computer program needs the power level at the cornea. This was found by taking the solar flux and calculating the power over the 7 mm pupil. The results from the program are

Retinal spot size	0.016 cm
Retinal heat flux	19.7 W/cm^2
Corneal heat flux	0.1 W/cm^2
Concentration ratio	1946

The image on the retina is much bigger than the image produced by a laser. An extended object cannot be focused down to as small a spot as a collimated beam. The heat flux on the retina is also much lower than for the lasers we have considered. Your knowledge about solar eclipses and staring at the Sun should convince you that even at 19.7 W/cm^2 the flux on the retina is dangerous. Remember that a flux level of approximately 2 W/cm^2 can burn paper. Paper does not have a cooling mechanism like the eye; however, you should never take chances.

EXAMPLE B.7

This example explores the dangers associated with getting too close to a 100 W light bulb. The power level is high compared to most of the continuous lasers studied in the foregoing examples. The difference is that the light bulb is an extended source and emits its power over 4 steradians. The properties of the bulb situation are

Source	Light bulb
Wavelength	Visible
Power level (cornea)	0.00031 W
Distance to object	1 m
Diameter of object	0.076 m (3 in.)

The power at the cornea was calculated by finding the surface of a sphere at the eye location from the bulb. The flux at this surface is found by dividing the power of the bulb by the surface area. The power at the cornea, for a 7 mm pupil, was found by multiplying the flux by the pupil area. The results from the program are

Retinal spot size	0.13 cm
Retinal heat flux	0.023 W/cm^2
Corneal heat flux	8.1 x 10^{-4} W/cm^2
Concentration ratio	28

The spot size on the retina is large in terms of our earlier examples. The heat flux is much lower than for the Sun. Integrated over time, this heat flux can lead to problems. Do not stare into any light source. Always take care of your eyes. They will not grow back.

We hope that this program is of use to you. Use it and become comfortable with its limitations and uses. Give it a try. Good luck!

TEACH.BAS

The computer program TEACH.BAS should also be useful to you. It is easy to execute and learn. This program was written to provide a tutorial for basic geometrical optics and a powerful lens matrix section for calculating the important aspects of lens systems.

Eleven basic lens systems are treated by this program. Lines 5700–6250 in the code describe the systems. You can choose to study any of these systems at one time, or you can have the program run through them all during one setting. You can adjust the speed of the presentation to quickly pass over certain sections that you learn to understand over time and get to the more difficult sections. The program provides a ray trace in color for each lens system and describes the image forming process.

Each lens system is clearly marked in the program code. The comments clearly mark the beginning of each section.

Concepts such as virtual images, field of view, and real image formation are covered in the program. Take a few minutes and give it a try. Even if you are an expert in optics you may find a user that can benefit from the program.

The second section contains the lens matrix program. This section begins on line 4585 in the program. A single lens or a large and complex system of lenses can be entered into the program for analysis. Stops and other nonimaging elements can be entered into the program. The program was delivered to you with the ability to handle five elements. The dimension statements in lines 46050 and 46100 can be changed, as needed, to provide for more system elements.

The program finds all the cardinal points for the lens system and many other important elements. The aperture stop for the system is also found along with the system pupils. Study the program and use it for several applications.

Now consider an example.

EXAMPLE B.8

Consider a three-lens system with an iris placed between lens 1 and 2. The lens system is being used to image an object 20 m away with a diameter of 1 m. The location of the image is needed along with the size and location of critical elements in the lens system.

Lens	Diameter	Focal Length	Distance to Next Object
#1	3 cm	10 cm	1 cm
Stop	1.5 cm	—	5 cm
#2	2 cm	5 cm	3 cm
#3	1 cm	-5 cm	—
Object	1 m (100 cm)	—	20 m to lens #1 (2000 cm)

The program output provides the following results:

    Effective focal length—4.8 cm

    Entrance pupil size and location—1.7 cm and 2000 cm from the object

Exit pupil size and location—1.5 cm and 4.3 cm from the image

Principal plane 1—0.58 cm to the right of lens 1

Principal plane 2—5.48 cm to the left of lens 3

Image location—4.82 cm from the second principal plane

This is a useful program that is easy to operate. Try several examples for yourself. Good hunting!

Program SAFETY.BAS

```
10 ' **** THIS IS PROGRAM SAFETY ****
20 KEY OFF
30 COLOR 15,1,1
40 SCREEN 0,1
50 WIDTH 80
60 CLS
70 PI=4*ATN(1!)
80 PRINT "DO YOU WANT THE LASER EYE SAFETY OR THE
   EYE MODEL PROGRAM?"
90 PRINT "ENTER E FOR THE EYE SAFETY OR M FOR THE
   EYE MODEL PROGRAM"
100 INPUT A$
110 IF A$="E" THEN GOTO 170
120 IF A$="e" THEN GOTO 170
130 IF A$="m" THEN GOTO 4420
140 IF A$="M" THEN GOTO 4420
150 PRINT "TRY AGAIN, YOUR ANSWER IS NOT USABLE"
160 GOTO 80
170 SPEED=2
180 SCREEN 1
190 COLOR 1,0
200 PRINT "               *"
```

```
210 PRINT "              ***"
220 PRINT "             *****"
230 PRINT "            *******"
240 PRINT "     THIS IS AN EYE SAFETY PROGRAM"
250 PRINT "IT WAS DEVELOPED FOR ENGINEERING OP-
    TICS"
260 PRINT "            *******"
270 PRINT "             *****"
280 PRINT "              ***"
290 PRINT "               *"
300 BB=1
310 GOSUB 4220
320 CLS
330 SCREEN 1
340 WIDTH 80
350 PRINT
    "*****************************************************************"
360 PRINT "*                                                       *"
370 PRINT "*      THIS PROGRAM PROVIDES CLASSIFICA-
    TIONS AND EXPOSURE LIMITS   *"
380 PRINT "*       FOR MOST COMMON LASERS.  FOR VIS-
    IBLE LASER BEAMS, THE    *"
390 PRINT "*        BLINK RESPONSE TIME (0.25 SECONDS) IS
    USED AS THE     *"
400 PRINT "*       MAXIMUM EXPOSURE TIME.  TEN SEC-
    ONDS IS USED AS THE      *"
410 PRINT "*       MAXIMUM EXPOSURE TIME FOR
    NONVISIBLE LASER BEAMS.     *"
420 PRINT "*                                                       *"
430 PRINT "*                   !! NOTE:!!                          *"
440 PRINT "*       THIS PROGRAM IS NOT A CERTIFIED
    LASER SAFETY PROGRAM.    *"
450 PRINT "*       THIS PROGRAM SHOULD BE USED FOR
    EDUCATIONAL PURPOSES.    *"
460 PRINT "*       THE EXPOSURE LIMITS AND LASER CLAS-
    SIFICATIONS GIVEN ARE   *"
470 PRINT "* TAKEN FROM ANSI Z136.1-1993 AND ARE
    CONSERVATIVE WHEN IN DOUBT. *"
480 PRINT
    "*****************************************************************"
490 PRINT " "
```

```
500 PRINT " "
510 PRINT "                    HIT SPACE BAR TO MOVE ON"
520 A$=INKEY$: IF A$="" THEN 520
530 GOTO 1110
540 CIRCLE (351,130),150,,.9*PI,1.1*PI,1
550 CIRCLE (65,130),150,,1.9*PI,.1*PI,1
560 LINE (208,50)-(208,210) 'vertical
570 LINE(0,130)-(320,130) 'horizontal
580 LINE (240,125)-(240,135),2 'back focus
590 LINE (176,125)-(176,135),2 'front focus
600 LINE (50,100)-(53,105),1 'arrow point
610 LINE (50,100)-(47,105),1 'arrow point
620 LINE (50,130)-(50,100),1 'object
630 BB=1: GOSUB 4250
640 LINE (50,100)-(70,100),1 'object
650 BB=1: GOSUB 4250
660 LINE (50,100)-(30,100),1 'object
670 BB=1: GOSUB 4250
680 LINE (50,100)-(50,80),1 'object
690 BB=1: GOSUB 4250
700 LINE (50,100)-(65,85),1 'object
710 BB=1: GOSUB 4250
720 LINE (50,100)-(35,85),1 'object
730 BB=1: GOSUB 4250
740 SPEED=1/5
750 CLS
760 GOSUB 4300
770 LINE (50,70)-(53,75),1 'arrow point
780 LINE (50,70)-(47,75),1 'arrow point
790 LINE (50,100)-(50,70),1 'object
800 PRINT "The tip of the extended object"
810 PRINT "can emit light in all directions."
820 BB=5: GOSUB 4250
830 LINE (50,70)-(70,70),1 'object
840 BB=2: GOSUB 4250
850 LINE (50,70)-(30,70),1 'object
860 BB=2: GOSUB 4250
870 LINE (50,70)-(50,50),1 'object
880 BB=2: GOSUB 4250
890 LINE (50,70)-(65,55),1 'object
```

```
900 BB=2: GOSUB 4250
910 LINE (50,70)-(35,55),1 'object
920 BB=5: GOSUB 4250
930 PRINT "But we are primarily interested"
940 PRINT "in just three specific light rays."
950 PRINT "These pass from the object to the"
960 FOR I=1 TO 8
970 PRINT ""
980 NEXT I
990 PRINT "lens.  One ray goes"
1000 PRINT "through one focus pt.,"
1010 PRINT "one goes through the"
1020 PRINT "vertex,and the last one"
1030 PRINT "goes through the other"
1040 PRINT "focus pt.  A collimated source sends"
1050 PRINT "all of them through the focal pt (at the retina)."
1060 BB=10: GOSUB 4250
1070 LINE (50,70)-(208,70) 'hori. trace
1080 LINE (208,70)-(293,150) 'focus trac
1090 LINE (50,70)-(290,116) 'vertex
1100 BB=10: GOSUB 4250
1110 CLS
1120 SCREEN 0,1
1130 WIDTH 80
1140 PRINT "Is the laser pulsed or continuous wave?"
1150 PRINT "Enter p or cw "
1160 INPUT LASER$
1170 PRINT "Enter the wavelength of the laser, micrometers "
1180 INPUT WAVE
1190 IF WAVE>100 THEN PRINT "THIS PROGRAM DOES NOT
     SUPPORT LASERS WITH WAVELENGTHS > THAN 100
     MICROMETERS"
1200 IF WAVE>100 THEN STOP
1210 IF LASER$="p" THEN GOTO 1250
1220 IF LASER$="P" THEN GOTO 1250
1230 IF LASER$="cw" THEN GOTO 2410
1240 IF LASER$="CW" THEN GOTO 2410
1250 PRINT "Enter the pulse duration (nanoseconds)"
1260 INPUT PTIME
1270 PRINT "Enter the pulse rate-PRF (per second-hz)"
1280 INPUT PRF
```

```
1290 PRINT "Enter the pulse energy (joules)"
1300 INPUT PENERGY
1310 PRINT "Enter beam diameter (in millimeters)"
1320 INPUT DIA
1330 AREA=PI/4*(DIA/10)^2   'change dia from mm to cm
1340 FLUX=PENERGY/AREA    'J/cm^2, the energy flux
1350 IF WAVE<.4001 THEN GOTO 1410
1360 IF WAVE<.7001 THEN GOTO 1510
1370 IF WAVE<1.06  THEN GOTO 1610
1380 IF WAVE<1.4  THEN GOTO 1710
1390 GOTO 1810
1400 '$$$$$$$$$$$$$$$$ PULSED LASERS $$$$$$$$$$$$$$$$$$$$$
1410
'********************************************************
1420 '        ULTRAVIOLET RANGE   0.2-0.4 MICROMETERS
1430
'********************************************************
1440 TYPE$="U"
1450 IF PENERGY<.0079 THEN CLASS=1
1460 IF PENERGY<.0079 THEN GOTO 1910
1470 IF FLUX<10 THEN CLASS=3
1480 IF FLUX<10 THEN GOTO 1910
1490 CLASS=4
1500 GOTO 1910
1510
'********************************************************
1520 '        VISIBLE RANGE   0.4-0.7 MICROMETERS
1530
'********************************************************
1540 TYPE$="V"
1550 IF PENERGY<.0000002 THEN CLASS=1
1560 IF PENERGY<.0000002 THEN GOTO 1910
1570 IF FLUX<.032 THEN CLASS=3
1580 IF FLUX<.032 THEN GOTO 1910
1590 CLASS=4
1600 GOTO 1910
1610
'********************************************************
1620 '        INFRARED RANGE   0.7-1.06 MICROMETERS
1630
'********************************************************
```

```
1640 TYPE$="I"
1650 IF PENERGY<.0000002 THEN CLASS=1
1660 IF PENERGY<.0000002 THEN GOTO 1910
1670 IF FLUX<.031 THEN CLASS=3
1680 IF FLUX<.031 THEN GOTO 1910
1690 CLASS=4
1700 GOTO 1910
1710
'**************************************************************
1720 '        INFRARED RANGE   1.06-1.4 MICROMETERS
1730
'**************************************************************
1740 TYPE$="I"
1750 IF PENERGY<.0000002 THEN CLASS=1
1760 IF PENERGY<.0000002 THEN GOTO 1910
1770 IF FLUX<.031 THEN CLASS=3
1780 IF FLUX<.031 THEN GOTO 1910
1790 CLASS=4
1800 GOTO 1910
1810
'**************************************************************
1820 '        FAR INFRARED RANGE   1.4-100 MICROMETERS
1830
'**************************************************************
1840 TYPE$="I"
1850 IF PENERGY<.01 THEN CLASS=1
1860 IF PENERGY<.01 THEN GOTO 1910
1870 IF FLUX<10 THEN CLASS=3
1880 IF FLUX<10 THEN GOTO 1910
1890 CLASS=4
1900 GOTO 1910
1910 CLS
1920 PRINT " "
1930 IF TYPE$="U" THEN PRINT
"**********************************************************
**************************** "
1940 IF TYPE$="U" THEN PRINT "   ULTRAVIOLET LASERS
PROVIDE CUMULATIVE EFFECTS FOR REPEATED
EXPOSURES."
1950 IF TYPE$="U" THEN PRINT "  FOR SAFE OPERATION,
```

```
REDUCE THE EL BY 2.5 IF REPETITIVE EXPOSURES"
1960 IF TYPE$="U" THEN PRINT "  ARE POSSIBLE OVER ANY
  24 HOUR PERIOD."
1970 IF TYPE$="V" THEN GOTO 2020
1980 IF TYPE$="I" THEN GOTO 2020
1990 PRINT " "
2000 PRINT "              HIT SPACE BAR TO CONTINUE"
2010 A$=INKEY$: IF A$="" THEN 2010
2020 CLS
2030 IF TYPE$="V" THEN TIM=.25
2040 IF TYPE$="I" THEN TIM=10!
2050 IF TYPE$="U" THEN TIM=10!
2060 N=PRF*TIM
2070 N=INT(N) 'N IS THE NUMBER OF PULSES DURING THE
  EXPOSURE
2080 CP=N^(-.25)
2090 IF PRF=1 THEN CP=1
2100 PRINT ""
2110 PRINT "*************************************************"
2120 PRINT "         LASER CLASSIFICATION"
2130 PRINT "*************************************************"
2140 PRINT " "
2150 PRINT "THESE ARE THE SPECIFICATIONS FOR YOUR
  LASER"
2160 PRINT " "
2170 PRINT "*** THIS IS A PULSED LASER ***"
2180 PRINT USING "THE LASER WAVELENGTH IS ##.####
  MICROMETERS";WAVE
2190 PRINT USING "THE ENERGY OUTPUT OF THE LASER IS
  ###.#### JOULES";PENERGY
2200 PRINT USING "THE ENERGY FLUX IS ######.###
  JOULES/CM^2";FLUX
2210 PRINT USING "THE PULSE REPETITION RATE IS ####/
  SECOND";PRF
2220 PRINT USING "THE BEAM DIAMETER IS ###
  MILLIMETERS";DIA
2230 PRINT USING "THE PULSE DURATION IS #########
  NANOSECONDS";PTIME
2240 PRINT " "
2250 PRINT "            ****            "
2260 PRINT USING "    THIS IS A CLASS ## DEVICE";CLASS
```

```
2270 PRINT "          ****          "
2280 PRINT " "
2290 GOSUB 3520
2300 PTIME=PTIME*E(9)
2310 EL=EL*10^-3
2320 EL=EL*CP
2330 PRINT USING "THE EXPOSURE LIMIT IS ##.##^^^^
     JOULES/CM^2 (NOTE ACTUAL ENERGY FLUX ABOVE)";EL
2340 PRINT USING "THE LIMITING APERTURE IS ## MM,
     AND CP= #.###";LA,CP
2350 PRINT USING "THE EXPOSURE TIME IS ##.##
     SECONDS";TIM
2360 PRINT "          ****          "
2370 PRINT "DO YOU WANT TO MAKE ANOTHER RUN? (1-
     YES, 0-NO)"
2380 INPUT RUNN
2390 IF RUNN=1 THEN GOTO 1110
2400 IF RUNN=0 THEN GOTO 3500
2410 '$$$$$$$$$$$$ CONTINUOUS WAVE LASERS
     $$$$$$$$$$$$
2420 PRINT "ENTER THE POWER OF THE LASER (WATTS)"
2430 INPUT POWER
2440 PRINT "ENTER THE BEAM DIAMETER (IN MILLIME-
     TERS)"
2450 INPUT DIA
2460 AREA=PI/4*(DIA/10)^2  'CHANGE DIA FROM MM TO CM
2470 FLUX=POWER/AREA   'W/cm2, HEAT FLUX
2480 IF WAVE<.4001 THEN GOTO 2530
2490 IF WAVE<.7001 THEN GOTO 2630
2500 IF WAVE<1.06  THEN GOTO 2750
2510 IF WAVE<1.4  THEN GOTO 2850
2520 GOTO 2950
2530
'*************************************************************
2540 '        ULTRAVIOLET RANGE   0.2-0.4 MICROMETERS
2550
'*************************************************************
2560 TYPE$="U"
2570 IF POWER<8E-10 THEN CLASS=1
2580 IF POWER<8E-10 THEN GOTO 3050
```

```
2590 IF POWER<.5 THEN CLASS=3
2600 IF POWER<.5 THEN GOTO 3050
2610 CLASS=4
2620 GOTO 3050
2630
'*********************************************************************
2640 '        VISIBLE RANGE   0.4-0.7 MICROMETERS
2650
'*********************************************************************
2660 TYPE$="V"
2670 IF POWER<.0000004 THEN CLASS=1
2680 IF POWER<.0000004 THEN GOTO 3050
2690 IF POWER<.001 THEN CLASS= 2
2700 IF POWER<.001 THEN GOTO 3050
2710 IF POWER<.5 THEN CLASS=3
2720 IF POWER<.5 THEN GOTO 3050
2730 CLASS=4
2740 GOTO 3050
2750
'*********************************************************************
2760 '        INFRARED RANGE   0.7-1.06 MICROMETERS
2770
'*********************************************************************
2780 TYPE$="I"
2790 IF POWER<.0000004 THEN CLASS=1
2800 IF POWER<.0000004 THEN GOTO 3050
2810 IF POWER<.5 THEN CLASS=3
2820 IF POWER<.5 THEN GOTO 3050
2830 CLASS=4
2840 GOTO 3050
2850
'*********************************************************************
2860 '        INFRARED RANGE   1.06-1.4 MICROMETERS
2870
'*********************************************************************
2880 TYPE$="I"
2890 IF POWER<.0002 THEN CLASS=1
2900 IF POWER<.0002 THEN GOTO 3050
2910 IF POWER<.5 THEN CLASS=3
2920 IF POWER<.5 THEN GOTO 3050
```

```
2930 CLASS=4
2940 GOTO 3050
2950
'******************************************************************
2960 '        FAR INFRARED RANGE   1.4-100 MICROMETERS
2970
'******************************************************************
2980 TYPE$="I"
2990 IF POWER<.0008 THEN CLASS=1
3000 IF POWER<.0008 THEN GOTO 3050
3010 IF POWER<.5 THEN CLASS=3
3020 IF POWER<.5 THEN GOTO 3050
3030 CLASS=4
3040 GOTO 3050
3050 CLS
3060 IF TYPE$="U" THEN PRINT " "
3070 IF TYPE$="U" THEN PRINT
"****************************************************************** "
3080 IF TYPE$="U" THEN PRINT "  ULTRAVIOLET LASERS
  PROVIDE CUMULATIVE EFFECTS FOR REPEATED EXPO-
  SURES."
3090 IF TYPE$="U" THEN PRINT "  FOR SAFE OPERATION,
  REDUCE THE EL BY 2.5 IF REPETITIVE EXPOSURES"
3100 IF TYPE$="U" THEN PRINT "  ARE POSSIBLE OVER ANY
  24 HOUR PERIOD."
3110 IF TYPE$="V" THEN GOTO 3160
3120 IF TYPE$="I" THEN GOTO 3160
3130 PRINT " "
3140 PRINT "                HIT SPACE BAR TO CONTINUE"
3150 A$=INKEY$: IF A$="" THEN 3150
3160 CLS
3170 PRINT " "
3180 PRINT "***********************************************"
3190 PRINT "        LASER CLASSIFICATION"
3200 PRINT "***********************************************"
3210 PRINT " "
3220 PRINT "THESE ARE THE SPECIFICATIONS FOR YOUR
  LASER"
3230 PTIME=10
3240 IF TYPE$="V" THEN PTIME=.25
3250 PRINT " "
```

```
3260 PRINT "*** THIS IS A CONTINUOUS WAVE LASER ***"
3270 PRINT USING "THE LASER WAVELENGTH IS ##.####
  MICROMETERS";WAVE
3280 PRINT USING "THE POWER OUTPUT OF THE LASER IS
  ###.#### WATTS";POWER
3290 PRINT USING "THE POWER FLUX IS ######.### WATTS/
  CM^2";FLUX
3300 EFLUX=FLUX*PTIME
3310 PRINT USING "THE ENERGY FLUX IS ##.###^^^^
  JOULES/CM^2";EFLUX
3320 PRINT USING "THE BEAM DIAMETER IS ###
  MILLIMETERS";DIA
3330 PRINT " "
3340 PRINT "            ****            "
3350 PRINT USING "    THIS IS A CLASS ## DEVICE";CLASS
3360 PRINT "            ****            "
3370 PRINT "  "
3380 PTIME=PTIME*10^(+9)
3390 GOSUB 3520
3400 EL=EL*10^-3
3410 PRINT USING "THE EXPOSURE LIMIT IS ##.##^^^^
  JOULES/CM^2 (NOTE ACTUAL ENERGY FLUX ABOVE)";EL
3420 PRINT USING "THE LIMITING APERTURE IS ## MM";LA
3430 IF PTIME=.25 THEN PRINT "THE EXPOSURE DURATION
  IS 0.25 SECONDS (BLINK RESPONSE)"
3440 IF PTIME=.25 GOTO 3460
3450 PRINT USING "THE EXPOSURE DURATION IS ##.##
  SECONDS ";PTIME
3460 PRINT " "
3470 PRINT "DO YOU WANT TO MAKE ANOTHER RUN? (1-
  YES, 0-NO)"
3480 INPUT RUNN
3490 IF RUNN=1 THEN GOTO 1110
3500 END
3510
'**************************************************************
3520 'EXPOSURE SUBROUTINE
3530
'**************************************************************
3540 PTIME=PTIME*10^(-9)
3550 LAMBDA=WAVE
```

```
3560 IF LAMBDA>.4 THEN GOTO 4020
3570 IF LAMBDA>.302 THEN 3600
3580 EL=3
3590 GOTO 3980
3600 IF LAMBDA>.303 THEN 3630
3610 EL=4
3620 GOTO 3980
3630 IF LAMBDA>.304 THEN 3660
3640 EL=6
3650 GOTO 3980
3660 IF LAMBDA>.305 THEN 3690
3670 EL=10
3680 GOTO 3980
3690 IF LAMBDA>.306 THEN 3720
3700 EL=16
3710 GOTO 3980
3720 IF LAMBDA>.307 THEN 3750
3730 EL=25
3740 GOTO 3980
3750 IF LAMBDA>.308 THEN 3780
3760 EL=40
3770 GOTO 3980
3780 IF LAMBDA>.309 THEN 3810
3790 EL=63
3800 GOTO 3980
3810 IF LAMBDA>.31 THEN 3840
3820 EL=100
3830 GOTO 3980
3840 IF LAMBDA>.311 THEN 3870
3850 EL=160
3860 GOTO 3980
3870 IF LAMBDA>.312 THEN 3900
3880 EL=250
3890 GOTO 3980
3900 IF LAMBDA>.313 THEN 3930
3910 EL=400
3920 GOTO 3980
3930 IF LAMBDA>.314 THEN GOTO 3960
3940 EL=630
3950 GOTO 3980
3960 IF LAMBDA>.4 THEN GOTO 4020
```

```
3970 EL=.56*(PTIME^.25)*1000
3980 EL1=.56*(PTIME^.25)*1000
3990 IF EL1<EL THEN EL=EL1
4000 LA=1
4010 RETURN
4020 IF LAMBDA>.7 THEN GOTO 4070
4030 IF PTIME<.000018 THEN EL=.0005
4040 IF PTIME<.000018 THEN GOTO 4200
4050 IF PTIME<10 THEN EL=1.8*PTIME^.75
4060 GOTO 4200
4070 IF LAMBDA>1.05 THEN GOTO 4120
4080 CA=10^(2*(LAMBDA-.7))
4090 IF PTIME<.000018 THEN EL=5*CA*.0001
4100 IF PTIME>=.000018 THEN EL=1.8*CA*PTIME^.75
4110 GOTO 4200
4120 IF LAMBDA>1.4 THEN GOTO 4160
4130 IF PTIME<.00005 THEN EL=.005
4140 IF PTIME>=.00005 THEN EL=9*PTIME^.75
4150 GOTO 4200
4160 IF PTIME<.0000001 THEN EL=10
4170 IF PTIME>=E-7 THEN EL=.56*PTIME^.25
4180 IF PTIME>10 THEN EL=.1
4190 IF PTIME>10 THEN PRINT "EL BECOMES FLUX"
4200 LA=7
4210 RETURN
4220 '
4230 'TIME DELAY SUBROUTINE
4240 '
4250 A=TIMER+(BB*SPEED)
4260 B=TIMER
4270 IF B>A THEN 4290
4280 GOTO 4260
4290 RETURN
4300 '
4310 'BASIC THIN LENS WITH AXIS
4320 '
4330 CIRCLE (351,100),150,,.9*PI,1.1*PI,1
4340 CIRCLE (65,100),150,,1.9*PI,.1*PI,1
4350 LINE (208,20)-(208,180) 'vertical
4360 LINE(0,100)-(320,100) 'horizontal
4370 LINE (240,95)-(240,105),2 'back focus
```

```
4380 LINE (176,95)-(176,105),2 'front focus
4390 RETURN
4400
'*****************************************************************
4410 'THIS PART OF THE PROGRAM MODELS THE EYE AND
     CALCULATES ENERGY AND HEAT
4420 'FLUXES ON THE CORNEA AND THE RETINA FOR
     LASERS AND EXTENDED SOURCES
4430
'*****************************************************************
4440 SCREEN 1
4450 COLOR 1,0
4460 PI=4*ATN(1!)
4470 CLS
4480 GOSUB 4300
4490 LINE (50,70)-(53,75),1 'arrow point
4500 LINE (50,70)-(47,75),1 'arrow point
4510 LINE (50,100)-(50,70),1 'object
4520 PRINT "An extended object"
4530 PRINT "can emit light in all directions."
4540 BB=5: GOSUB 4250
4550 LINE (50,70)-(70,70),1 'object
4560 BB=2: GOSUB 4250
4570 LINE (50,70)-(30,70),1 'object
4580 BB=2: GOSUB 4250
4590 LINE (50,70)-(50,50),1 'object
4600 BB=2: GOSUB 4250
4610 LINE (50,70)-(65,55),1 'object
4620 BB=2: GOSUB 4250
4630 LINE (50,70)-(35,55),1 'object
4640 BB=5: GOSUB 4250
4650 PRINT "But a laser emits collimated"
4660 PRINT "light rays."
4670 FOR I=1 TO 9
4680 PRINT ""
4690 NEXT I
4700 PRINT "This program is an"
4710 PRINT "approximation to the "
4720 PRINT "optical functions of "
4730 PRINT "the eye using the thin "
4740 PRINT "lens eq. and diffraction"
```

```
4750 PRINT "limited operation."
4760 BB=10: GOSUB 4250
4770 LINE (208,70)-(50,70) 'focus trac
4780 LINE (208,70)-(293,150) 'focus trac
4790 LINE (50,70)-(290,116) 'vertex
4800 PRINT ""
4810 PRINT ""
4820 PRINT "HIT SPACE BAR TO CONTINUE"
4830 A$=INKEY$: IF A$="" THEN 4830
4840 CLS
4850 SCREEN 0,1
4860 WIDTH 80
4870 PI=4*ATN(1)
4880 PRINT
     "******************************************************** "
4890 B$="THIS PROGRAM IS A SIMPLE APPROXIMATION TO
     THE OPTICAL FUNCTIONS OF THE EYE"
4900 A$="    DO NOT TAKE THESE NUMBERS AS ANY MORE
     THAN AN EDUCATIONAL EXERCISE"
4910 PRINT B$
4920 PRINT A$
4930 PI=4*ATN(1)
4940 NLENS=1
4950 PRINT " "
4960 PRINT "*********************** THIN LENS APPROXIMA-
     TION FOR THE EYE *******************"
4970 PRINT " "
4980 SOURCE=0
4990 F=1.7   'EFFECTIVE FOCAL LENGTH FOR EYE, CM
5000 INPUT "IS THE SOURCE A LASER OR AN EXTENDED
     OBJECT? (L FOR LASER, E FOR EXT. OBJECT)";SOURCE$
5010 IF SOURCE$="L" THEN SOURCE=1
5020 IF SOURCE$="l" THEN SOURCE=1
5030 IF SOURCE=1 THEN INPUT "WHAT IS THE POWER OF
     THE LASER? (WATTS) ";POWER
5040 IF SOURCE=1 THEN INPUT "WHAT IS THE WAVE-
     LENGTH OF THE LASER? (MICROMETERS) ";LAMBDA
5050 IF SOURCE=1 THEN GOTO 5120
5060 INPUT "POWER FROM OBJECT ON CORNEA, (WATTS,
     FOR A PUPIL SIZE OF 7 MM)";POWER
5070 INPUT "INPUT DISTANCE TO OBJECT (METERS) ";SO
```

```
5080 INPUT "INPUT DIAMETER OF OBJECT (METERS) ";DIA
5090 SOC=SO*100
5100 SI=1/(1/F-1/SOC)/100
5110 GOTO 5150
5120 INPUT "INPUT DIAMETER OF LASER BEAM (MM) ";DIA
5130 IF SOURCE=1 THEN SI=.017
5140 DIA=DIA/1000    'CONVERT LASER BEAM DIA TO
  METERS
5150 CLS
5160 PRINT " "
5170 PRINT
  "*********************************************************** "
5180 PRINT " "
5190 PRINT "        THIS PROGRAM CALCULATES THE CON-
  CENTRATION ON THE RETINA "
5200 PRINT "        AND THE HEAT FLUX ON THE RETINA
  FOR THE IDEAL EYE"
5210 PRINT " "
5220 PRINT USING " THE EFFECTIVE FOCAL LENGTH IS =
  ###.### CM";F
5230 IF SOURCE=1 THEN GOTO 5280
5240 PRINT USING " THE OBJECT IS LOCATED ##.###^^^^ M
  FROM THE EYE";SO
5250 PRINT USING " THE DIAMETER OF THE OBJECT IS
  ##.###^^^^ M ";DIA
5260 PRINT USING " THE POWER FROM THE OBJECT AT
  THE CORNEA IS ####.### W ";POWER
5270 GOTO 5300
5280 PRINT USING " THE DIAMETER OF THE LASER BEAM
  IS ###.### MM ";DIA*1000
5290 PRINT USING " THE POWER FROM THE LASER IS
  ####.##### W ";POWER
5300 PRINT " "
5310 SET=0
5320 IF SOURCE=0 THEN LAMBDA=.56   'REFERENCE WAVE-
  LENGTH FOR EXTENDED SOURCE
5330 D=1.22*(F/100*LAMBDA/1000000!/DIA)*2   'DIFFRACTION
  LIMIT DIAMETER, M
5340 IF SOURCE=0 THEN M=-SI/SO   'MAGNIFICATION FOR
  EXTENDED SOURCE
5350 IF SOURCE=0 THEN IMAGE=-M*DIA   'IMAGE DIAM-
  ETER, M
```

5360 IF SOURCE=1 THEN IMAGE=DIA/316.23   'IMAGE DIAM-
ETER, M
5370 IF D>IMAGE THEN SET=1
5380 IF D>IMAGE THEN IMAGE=D 'DO NOT LET DIA BE
SMALLER THAN DIFFRACTION LIMIT
5390 IF SOURCE=1 THEN M=-IMAGE/DIA 'MAGNIFICATION
FOR DIFFRACTION LIMITED CASE
5400 PRINT USING " THE MAGNIFICATION IS ##.###^^^^";M
5410 IF SET=1 THEN PRINT USING " THE SPOT SIZE ON THE
RETINA IS ##.###^^^^ CM (DIFFRACTION
LIMITED)";IMAGE*100
5420 IF SET=0 THEN PRINT USING " THE SPOT SIZE ON THE
RETINA IS ##.###^^^^ CM ";IMAGE*100
5430 AREA=PI/4*IMAGE^2*10000 'RETINAL IMAGE OF OB-
JECT
5440 FLUX=POWER/AREA   'HEAT FLUX ON RETINA, W/CM^2
5450 IF SOURCE=0 THEN DIA=.007   'USE PUPIL AREA FOR
EXTENDED OBJECT
5460 FLUXC=POWER/(PI/4*DIA*DIA)/10000 'FLUX AT COR-
NEA, W/CM^2
5470 PRINT USING " THE HEAT FLUX ON THE RETINA IS
##.###^^^^ W/CM^2";FLUX
5480 PRINT USING " THE HEAT FLUX ON THE CORNEA IS
##.###^^^^ W/CM^2";FLUXC
5490 CONCEN=FLUX/FLUXC
5500 PRINT USING " THE CONCENTRATION RATIO, RELA-
TIVE TO THE FLUX ON THE CORNEA IS, ######";CONCEN
5510 IF SET=0 THEN PRINT USING " THE DIFFRACTION
LIMITED IMAGE SIZE IS ##.###^^^^ CM ";D*100
5520 PRINT " "
5530 PRINT "*** A CLASS II VISIBLE LASER HAS A MAXIMUM
POWER OF 1 mW AT THE CORNEA ***"
5540 PRINT "   *************** REMEMBER ****************"
5550 PRINT " THE DIAMETER OF THE MACULA LUTEA IS 0.3
CM. COMPARE THIS TO YOUR IMAGE SIZE."
5560 END

Program TEACH.BAS

```
25 ' **** THIS IS PROGRAM TEACH ****
50 KEY OFF
100 SCREEN 0,1
150 WIDTH 80
200 CLS
250 PRINT "DO YOU WANT THE TUTORIAL OR THE LENS
   MATRIX PROGRAM?"
300 PRINT "ENTER T FOR THE TUTORIAL OR M FOR THE
   LENS MATRIX PROGRAM"
350 INPUT A$
400 IF A$="T" THEN GOTO 700
450 IF A$="t" THEN GOTO 700
500 IF A$="m" THEN GOTO 45850
550 IF A$="M" THEN GOTO 45850
600 PRINT "TRY AGAIN, YOUR ANSWER IS NOT USABLE"
650 GOTO 250
700 SPEED=1
750 PI=4*ATN(1!)
800 SCREEN 1
850 COLOR 0,1
900 'SPEED=1/10
950 'GOTO 39100
1000 PRINT "            *"
1050 PRINT "           ***"
1100 PRINT "          *****"
1150 PRINT "         *******"
1200 PRINT " THIS IS A TUTORIAL RAY TRACE PROGRAM"
1250 PRINT "IT WAS DEVELOPED FOR ENGINEERING OP-
   TICS"
1300 PRINT "         *******"
1350 PRINT "          *****"
1400 PRINT "           ***"
1450 PRINT "            *"
1500 CIRCLE (351,130),150,,.9*PI,1.1*PI,1
1550 CIRCLE (65,130),150,,1.9*PI,.1*PI,1
1600 LINE (208,50)-(208,210) 'vertical
1650 LINE(0,130)-(320,130) 'horizontal
1700 LINE (240,125)-(240,135),2 'back focus
1750 LINE (176,125)-(176,135),2 'front focus
```

```
1800 LINE (50,100)-(53,105),1 'arrow point
1850 LINE (50,100)-(47,105),1 'arrow point
1900 LINE (50,130)-(50,100),1 'object
1950 BB=1: GOSUB 41300
2000 LINE (50,100)-(70,100),1 'object
2050 BB=1: GOSUB 41300
2100 LINE (50,100)-(30,100),1 'object
2150 BB=1: GOSUB 41300
2200 LINE (50,100)-(50,80),1 'object
2250 BB=1: GOSUB 41300
2300 LINE (50,100)-(65,85),1 'object
2350 BB=1: GOSUB 41300
2400 LINE (50,100)-(35,85),1 'object
2450 BB=1: GOSUB 41300
2500 CLS
2550 PRINT "SET DISPLAY SPEED"
2600 PRINT "INPUT 1 FOR AVERAGE SPEED"
2650 PRINT "INPUT A NUMBER >1 FOR FASTER SPEED"
2700 PRINT "INPUT A NUMBER <1 FOR SLOWER SPEED"
2750 INPUT SPEED
2800 SPEED=1/SPEED
2850 CLS
2900 GOSUB 41550
2950 LINE (50,70)-(53,75),1 'arrow point
3000 LINE (50,70)-(47,75),1 'arrow point
3050 LINE (50,100)-(50,70),1 'object
3100 PRINT "The tip of the object point"
3150 PRINT "can emit light in all directions."
3200 BB=5: GOSUB 41300
3250 LINE (50,70)-(70,70),1 'object
3300 BB=2: GOSUB 41300
3350 LINE (50,70)-(30,70),1 'object
3400 BB=2: GOSUB 41300
3450 LINE (50,70)-(50,50),1 'object
3500 BB=2: GOSUB 41300
3550 LINE (50,70)-(65,55),1 'object
3600 BB=2: GOSUB 41300
3650 LINE (50,70)-(35,55),1 'object
3700 BB=5: GOSUB 41300
3750 PRINT "But we are primarily interested"
```

```
3800 PRINT "in just three specific light rays."
3850 PRINT "These pass from the object to the"
3900 FOR I=1 TO 8
3950 PRINT ""
4000 NEXT I
4050 PRINT "lens.  One ray goes"
4100 PRINT "through one focus pt.,"
4150 PRINT "one goes through the"
4200 PRINT "vertex,and the last one"
4250 PRINT "goes through the other"
4300 PRINT "focus pt.  We will use two of these."
4350 PRINT "All of them will cross at the image pt."
4400 BB=10: GOSUB 41300
4450 LINE (50,70)-(208,70) 'hori. trace
4500 LINE (208,70)-(293,150) 'focus trac
4550 LINE (50,70)-(290,116) 'vertex
4600 BB=10: GOSUB 41300
4650 CLS
4700 PRINT "RESET DISPLAY SPEED(if desired)"
4750 PRINT "INPUT 1 FOR AVERAGE SPEED"
4800 PRINT "INPUT A NUMBER >1 FOR FASTER SPEED"
4850 PRINT "INPUT A NUMBER <1 FOR SLOWER SPEED"
4900 PRINT "INPUT RETURN TO KEEP PREVIOUS FACTOR"
4950 INPUT SPEE
5000 IF SPEE=0 THEN GOTO 5100
5050 SPEED=1/SPEE
5100 CLS
5150 PRINT "you can choose to see all of the ray traces or any one
     of them"
5200 PRINT ""
5250 PRINT "do you want to see all of the ray traces? (0-no, 1-yes,
     2-stop) "
5300 INPUT ANS
5350 IF ANS=2 THEN GOTO 41100
5400 IF ANS=1 THEN GOTO 7200
5450 IF ANS=0 THEN GOTO 5700
5500 CLS
5550 PRINT "YOUR RESPONSE IS NOT USABLE, TRY AGAIN"
5600 PRINT " "
5650 GOTO 5150
5700 PRINT " the available ray traces are"
```

```
5750 PRINT "1-single lens, far object"
5800 PRINT "2-single lens, object at 2f"
5850 PRINT "3-single lens, object at 1.5f"
5900 PRINT "4-single lens, object at f"
5950 PRINT "5-single lens, object at 0.5f"
6000 PRINT "6-negative thin lens, far object"
6050 PRINT "7-negative thin lens, object at 1.5f"
6100 PRINT "8-two lens system, far object"
6150 PRINT "9-two lens system, far object, #2"
6200 PRINT "10-two lens system, one negative lens"
6250 PRINT "11-two lens system, field of view"
6300 PRINT "choose one "
6350 INPUT CHOICE
6400 IF CHOICE=1 THEN GOTO 7200
6450 IF CHOICE=2 THEN GOTO 9850
6500 IF CHOICE=3 THEN GOTO 13000
6550 IF CHOICE=4 THEN GOTO 15950
6600 IF CHOICE=5 THEN GOTO 19100
6650 IF CHOICE=6 THEN GOTO 22750
6700 IF CHOICE=7 THEN GOTO 25750
6750 IF CHOICE=8 THEN GOTO 28900
6800 IF CHOICE=9 THEN GOTO 32350
6850 IF CHOICE=10 THEN GOTO 35800
6900 IF CHOICE=11 THEN GOTO 39150
6950 CLS
7000 PRINT "YOUR RESPONSE IS NOT USABLE, TRY AGAIN"
7050 PRINT " "
7100 GOTO 5150
7150 '******** THIS IS EXAMPLE #1 ********
7200 CLS
7250 PRINT ""
7300 PRINT "**THIS IS A SIMPLE THIN LENS EXAMPLE**"
7350 PRINT ""
7400 PRINT "THE OBJECT IS SEVERAL FOCAL LENGTHS
  FROM THE LENS"
7450 PRINT "NOTE THAT THE IMAGE WILL BE MINIMIZED
  AND INVERTED"
7500 PRINT ""
7550 PRINT "          ************"
7600 PRINT "     THE THIN LENS EQUATION IS"
7650 PRINT "        1/Xo + 1/Xi = 1/f"
```

```
7700 PRINT ""
7750 PRINT " FOR THIS CASE Xo IS SEVERAL TIMES f, OR"
7800 PRINT "          Xo=mf, m>>1"
7850 PRINT ""
7900 PRINT "     Xi = (1-m)f, REAL IMAGE"
7950 PRINT ""
8000 PRINT "   THE MAGNIFICATION IS -Xi/Xo, OR"
8050 PRINT "        MAG = -((1-m)/m)"
8100 PRINT ""
8150 PRINT "MAG IS NEGATIVE, HENCE AN INVERTED
  IMAGE"
8200 'BB=25: GOSUB 6750
8250 LOCATE 25,1
8300 PRINT "HIT SPACE BAR TO MOVE ON"
8350 A$=INKEY$: IF A$="" THEN 8350
8400 LOCATE 25,1
8450 PRINT ""
8500 CLS
8550 GOSUB 41700
8600 LINE (0,100)-(0,70),1 'object
8650 LINE (0,70)-(3,75),1 'arrow point
8700 PRINT "object ray appears to come from infinity as it hits the
  lens"
8750 BB=5: GOSUB 41300
8800 LINE (0,70)-(208,70) 'hori. trace
8850 PRINT "the lens forces this ray through the back focal point"
8900 BB=5: GOSUB 41300
8950 LINE (208,70)-(293,150) 'focus trace
9000 PRINT "next a ray from the object passes through the vertex"
9050 BB=5: GOSUB 41300
9100 LINE (0,70)-(320,116) 'vertex
9150 FOR I=1 TO 9
9200 PRINT ""
9250 NEXT I
9300 PRINT "the image is formed"
9350 PRINT "behind the lens where"
9400 PRINT "the rays cross"
9450 LINE (245,100)-(245,105),2 'image
9500 CIRCLE (245,100),10,2,,,1
9550 LOCATE 25,1
9600 PRINT "HIT SPACE BAR TO MOVE ON"
```

```
9650 A$=INKEY$: IF A$="" THEN 9650
9700 CLS
9750 IF ANS=0 THEN GOTO 4650
9800 '******** THIS IS EXAMPLE #2 ********
9850 CLS
9900 LOCATE 25,1
9950 PRINT "HIT SPACE BAR TO MOVE ON"
10000 PRINT "**NOW TAKE THE OBJECT TO 2F, OR TWO
  TIMES THE FOCAL LENGTH**"
10050 PRINT ""
10100 PRINT "NOTE THAT THE IMAGE IS INVERTED, BUT
  NO MAGNIFICATION"
10150 PRINT""
10200 PRINT"          ************"
10250 PRINT "      THE THIN LENS EQUATION IS"
10300 PRINT "          1/Xo + 1/Xi = 1/f
10350 PRINT ""
10400 PRINT "  FOR THIS CASE Xo IS TWO TIMES f, OR"
10450 PRINT "           Xo=2f "
10500 PRINT ""
10550 PRINT "       Xi = 2f, REAL IMAGE"
10600 PRINT ""
10650 PRINT "   THE MAGNIFICATION IS -Xi/Xo, OR"
10700 PRINT "          MAG = -1"
10750 PRINT ""
10800 PRINT "MAG IS NEGATIVE, HENCE AN INVERTED
  IMAGE"
10850 PRINT ""
10900 PRINT ""
10950 'BB=25: GOSUB 6750
11000 A$=INKEY$: IF A$="" THEN 11000
11050 LOCATE 25,1
11100 PRINT ""
11150 CLS
11200 '
11250 '****** NOW DO 2F EXAMPLE ********
11300 '
11350 GOSUB 41700
11400 LINE (142,100)-(142,70),1 'object
11450 LINE (142,70)-(145,75),1 'arrow point
11500 LINE (142,70)-(139,75),1 'arrow point
```

```
11550 LINE (142,95)-(142,105),2 'forward 2f
11600 LINE (272,95)-(272,105),2 'back 2f
11650 PRINT "object ray appears to come from infinity as it hits
   the lens"
11700 BB=5: GOSUB 41300
11750 LINE (142,70)-(208,70) 'hori. trace
11800 PRINT "the lens forces this ray through the back focal point"
11850 BB=5: GOSUB 41300
11900 LINE (208,70)-(293,150) 'focus trac
11950 PRINT "next a ray from the object passes through the
   vertex"
12000 BB=5: GOSUB 41300
12050 LINE (142,70)-(318,150) 'vertex
12100 LINE (272,100)-(272,130),2 'image
12150 CIRCLE (272,130),10,2,,,1
12200 FOR I=1 TO 9
12250 PRINT ""
12300 NEXT I
12350 PRINT"NOTE: THE IMAGE IS THE"
12400 PRINT"SAME DISTANCE FROM THE"
12450 PRINT"LENS AS THE OBJECT, BUT"
12500 PRINT"IN THE IMAGE SPACE.  ALSO"
12550 PRINT"NOTE THAT THE MAGNIFICATION"
12600 PRINT"IS -1."
12650 LOCATE 25,1
12700 PRINT "HIT SPACE BAR TO MOVE ON"
12750 A$=INKEY$: IF A$="" THEN 12750
12800 'BB=15: GOSUB 7450
12850 CLS
12900 IF ANS=0 THEN GOTO 4650
12950 '******** THIS IS EXAMPLE #3 ********
13000 CLS
13050 LOCATE 25,1
13100 PRINT "HIT SPACE BAR TO MOVE ON"
13150 PRINT "**NOW LET THE OBJECT MOVE TO 1.5F **"
13200 PRINT ""
13250 PRINT "NOTE THAT THE IMAGE WILL BE MAGNIFIED,
   INVERTED, AND REAL"
13300 PRINT""
13350 PRINT"          ************"
13400 PRINT "    THE THIN LENS EQUATION IS"
```

```
13450 PRINT "        1/Xo + 1/Xi = 1/f
13500 PRINT ""
13550 PRINT "  FOR THIS CASE Xo IS 1.5 TIMES f, OR"
13600 PRINT "          Xo=1.5f "
13650 PRINT ""
13700 PRINT "        Xi = 3f, REAL IMAGE"
13750 PRINT ""
13800 PRINT "    THE MAGNIFICATION IS -Xi/Xo, OR"
13850 PRINT "          MAG = -2"
13900 PRINT ""
13950 PRINT "MAG IS NEGATIVE, HENCE AN INVERTED
   IMAGE"
14000 PRINT ""
14050 PRINT ""
14100 PRINT ""
14150 'BB=25: GOSUB 6750
14200 A$=INKEY$: IF A$="" THEN 14200
14250 LOCATE 25,1
14300 PRINT ""
14350 CLS
14400 GOSUB 41700
14450 LINE (142,95)-(142,105),2 'forward 2f
14500 LINE (272,95)-(272,105),2 'back 2f
14550 LINE (159,100)-(159,70),1 'object
14600 LINE (159,70)-(163,75),1 'arrow point
14650 LINE (159,70)-(155,75),1 'arrow point
14700 PRINT "object ray appears to come from infinity as it hits
   the lens"
14750 BB=5: GOSUB 41300
14800 LINE (159,70)-(208,70) 'hori. trac
14850 PRINT "the lens forces this ray through the back focal point"
14900 BB=5: GOSUB 41300
14950 LINE (208,70)-(309,165) 'focus tra
15000 PRINT "next a ray from the object passes through the
   vertex"
15050 BB=5: GOSUB 41300
15100 LINE (159,70)-(306,160) 'vertex
15150 FOR I=1 TO 9
15200 PRINT ""
15250 NEXT I
15300 LINE (300,100)-(300,157),2 'image
```

```
15350 CIRCLE (300,157),10,2,,,1
15400 PRINT "the image is greatly"
15450 PRINT "magnified, but still"
15500 PRINT "located on the image side"
15550 PRINT "of the lens. The image is real."
15600 LOCATE 25,1
15650 PRINT "HIT SPACE BAR TO MOVE ON"
15700 A$=INKEY$: IF A$="" THEN 15700
15750 'BB=15: GOSUB 7450
15800 CLS
15850 IF ANS=0 THEN GOTO 4650
15900 '******** THIS IS EXAMPLE #4 ********
15950 CLS
16000 LOCATE 25,1
16050 PRINT "HIT SPACE BAR TO MOVE ON"
16100 PRINT "   **NOW LET THE OBJECT MOVE TO F**"
16150 PRINT ""
16200 PRINT "NOTE THAT THE IMAGE WILL BE AT INFIN-
      ITY"
16250 PRINT""
16300 PRINT"          ************"
16350 PRINT "     THE THIN LENS EQUATION IS"
16400 PRINT "        1/Xo + 1/Xi = 1/f
16450 PRINT ""
16500 PRINT " FOR THIS CASE Xo IS EQUAL TO f, OR"
16550 PRINT "            Xo=f "
16600 PRINT ""
16650 PRINT "       Xi = 1/0, INFINITY!!"
16700 PRINT ""
16750 PRINT "  THE MAGNIFICATION IS -Xi/Xo, OR"
16800 PRINT "        MAG = INFINITE"
16850 PRINT ""
16900 PRINT ""
16950 PRINT ""
17000 PRINT ""
17050 PRINT ""
17100 'BB=20: GOSUB 6750
17150 A$=INKEY$: IF A$="" THEN 17150
17200 LOCATE 25,1
17250 PRINT ""
17300 CLS
```

```
17350 GOSUB 41700
17400 LINE (142,95)-(142,105),2 'forward 2f
17450 LINE (272,95)-(272,105),2 'back 2f
17500 LINE (176,100)-(176,70),1 'object
17550 LINE (176,70)-(181,75),1 'arrow point
17600 LINE (176,70)-(171,75),1 'arrow point
17650 PRINT "object ray appears to come from infinity as it hits
   the lens"
17700 BB=5: GOSUB 41300
17750 LINE (176,70)-(208,70) 'hori. trac
17800 BB=5: GOSUB 41300
17850 PRINT "the lens forces this ray through the back focal point"
17900 BB=5: GOSUB 41300
17950 LINE (208,70)-(309,165) 'focus tra
18000 PRINT "next a ray from the object passes through the
   vertex"
18050 BB=5: GOSUB 41300
18100 LINE (176,70)-(272,160) 'vertex
18150 FOR I=1 TO 9
18200 PRINT ""
18250 NEXT I
18300 BB=10: GOSUB 41300
18350 PRINT "The rays never"
18400 PRINT "cross.  An object"
18450 PRINT "at the focal pt."
18500 PRINT "gives an image at"
18550 PRINT "infinity."
18600 LOCATE 25,1
18650 PRINT "HIT SPACE BAR TO MOVE ON"
18700 A$=INKEY$: IF A$="" THEN 18700
18750 'BB=15: GOSUB 7450
18800 CLS
18850 IF ANS=0 THEN GOTO 4650
18900 '
18950 '*** MOVE TO 0.5F ***
19000 '
19050 '******** THIS IS EXAMPLE #5 ********
19100 CLS
19150 LOCATE 25,1
19200 PRINT "HIT SPACE BAR TO MOVE ON"
19250 PRINT ""
```

```
19300 PRINT "**NOW THE OBJECT WILL MOVE TO 0.5F**"
19350 PRINT ""
19400 PRINT "NOTE THAT THE IMAGE WILL BE MAGNIFIED,
      ERECT, AND VIRTUAL"
19450 PRINT ""
19500 PRINT"         ************"
19550 PRINT "     THE THIN LENS EQUATION IS"
19600 PRINT "        1/Xo + 1/Xi = 1/f
19650 PRINT ""
19700 PRINT "  FOR THIS CASE Xo IS 0.5 TIMES f, OR"
19750 PRINT "            Xo=0.5f "
19800 PRINT ""
19850 PRINT "    Xi = -f, VIRTUAL IMAGE!!"
19900 PRINT ""
19950 PRINT "   THE MAGNIFICATION IS -Xi/Xo, OR"
20000 PRINT "          MAG = 2"
20050 PRINT ""
20100 PRINT " MAG IS POSITIVE, HENCE AN ERECT IMAGE"
20150 PRINT ""
20200 PRINT ""
20250 PRINT ""
20300 'BB=25: GOSUB 6750
20350 A$=INKEY$: IF A$="" THEN 20350
20400 LOCATE 25,1
20450 PRINT ""
20500 CLS
20550 GOSUB 41700
20600 LINE (142,95)-(142,105),2 'forward 2f
20650 LINE (272,95)-(272,105),2 'back 2f
20700 LINE (193,100)-(193,70),1 'object
20750 LINE (193,70)-(188,75),1 'arrow point
20800 LINE (193,70)-(198,75),1 'arrow point
20850 PRINT "object ray appears to come from infinity as it hits
      the lens"
20900 BB=5: GOSUB 41300
20950 LINE (193,70)-(208,70) 'hori. trac
21000 BB=5: GOSUB 41300
21050 FOR I=1 TO 2
21100 PRINT ""
21150 NEXT I
21200 PRINT "the lens forces the"
```

```
21250 PRINT "ray through the back"
21300 PRINT "focal pt."
21350 PRINT ""
21400 BB=5: GOSUB 41300
21450 LINE (208,70)-(309,165) 'focus tra
21500 LINE (208,70)-(135,0) 'focus tra
21550 PRINT "next a ray from the"
21600 PRINT "object passes through"
21650 PRINT "the vertex"
21700 BB=5: GOSUB 41300
21750 LINE (193,70)-(243,170),1 'vertex
21800 LINE (193,70)-(154,0),1 'vertex
21850 LINE (176,100)-(176,39),1 'image
21900 CIRCLE (176,40),10,2,,,1
21950 PRINT ""
22000 PRINT ""
22050 PRINT ""
22100 PRINT "the rays diverge on the"
22150 PRINT "image side of the lens."
22200 PRINT "The image shows up on"
22250 PRINT "the object side of the"
22300 PRINT "lens as a magnified,"
22350 PRINT "erect, and virtual image"
22400 LOCATE 25,1
22450 PRINT "HIT SPACE BAR TO MOVE ON"
22500 A$=INKEY$: IF A$="" THEN 22500
22550 ' BB=15: GOSUB 7450
22600 CLS
22650 IF ANS=0 THEN GOTO 4650
22700 '******** THIS IS EXAMPLE #6 ********
22750 CLS
22800 LOCATE 25,1
22850 PRINT "HIT SPACE BAR TO MOVE ON"
22900 PRINT "**THIS IS A NEGATIVE THIN LENS EX-
      AMPLE**"
22950 PRINT ""
23000 PRINT "NOTE THAT THE IMAGE WILL ALWAYS BE
      ERECT, MINIFIED, AND VIRTUAL FOR A NEGATIVE LENS"
23050 PRINT "        ************"
23100 PRINT "     THE THIN LENS EQUATION IS"
23150 PRINT "        1/Xo + 1/Xi = 1/-f "
```

```
23200 PRINT ""
23250 PRINT "FOR THIS CASE Xo IS SEVERAL TIMES f, OR"
23300 PRINT "          Xo=mf, m>>f "
23350 PRINT ""
23400 PRINT "  Xi = -(m/(1+m))f, VIRTUAL IMAGE!!"
23450 PRINT ""
23500 PRINT "   THE MAGNIFICATION IS -Xi/Xo, OR"
23550 PRINT "         MAG = 1/(1+m)"
23600 PRINT ""
23650 PRINT " MAG IS POSITIVE, HENCE AN ERECT IMAGE"
23700 PRINT ""
23750 PRINT " -f IS USED IN THE THIN LENS EQUATION"
23800 PRINT "  BECAUSE A NEGATIVE THIN LENS HAS A"
23850 PRINT "      NEGATIVE FOCAL LENGTH"
23900 'BB=25: GOSUB 6750
23950 A$=INKEY$: IF A$="" THEN 23950
24000 LOCATE 25,1
24050 PRINT ""
24100 CLS
24150 GOSUB 42050
24200 LINE (0,100)-(0,70),1 'object
24250 LINE (0,70)-(4,75),1 'arrow point
24300 PRINT "object ray appears to come from infinity as it hits
      the lens"
24350 BB=5: GOSUB 41300
24400 LINE (0,70)-(208,70) 'hori. trac
24450 PRINT "the lens forces this ray to diverge as if it came from
      the front focus"
24500 BB=5: GOSUB 41300
24550 PRINT "next a ray from the object passes through the
      vertex"
24600 LINE (176,100)-(249,30) 'focus tra
24650 BB=5: GOSUB 41300
24700 LINE (0,70)-(300,113) 'vertex
24750 BB=5: GOSUB 41300
24800 FOR I=1 TO 8
24850 PRINT ""
24900 NEXT I
24950 LINE (180,100)-(180,96),2 'image
25000 CIRCLE (180,96),10,2,,,1
25050 PRINT "the image is minified"
```

```
25100 PRINT "erect and virtual"
25150 PRINT ""
25200 PRINT "NOTE: THE VIRTUAL"
25250 PRINT "IMAGE IS ALWAYS BETWEEN"
25300 PRINT "THE FRONT FOCUS AND THE"
25350 PRINT "LENS FOR A NEGATIVE LENS"
25400 LOCATE 25,1
25450 PRINT "HIT SPACE BAR TO MOVE ON"
25500 A$=INKEY$: IF A$="" THEN 25500
25550 'BB=15: GOSUB 7450
25600 CLS
25650 IF ANS=0 THEN GOTO 4650
25700 '******** THIS IS EXAMPLE #7 ********
25750 CLS
25800 LOCATE 25,1
25850 PRINT "HIT SPACE BAR TO MOVE ON"
25900 PRINT "**THIS IS A NEGATIVE THIN LENS EX-
   AMPLE**"
25950 PRINT ""
26000 PRINT "NOTE THAT THE IMAGE WILL ALWAYS BE
   ERECT, MINIFIED, AND VIRTUAL FOR A NEGATIVE LENS"
26050 PRINT"        ************"
26100 PRINT "     THE THIN LENS EQUATION IS"
26150 PRINT "        1/Xo + 1/Xi = 1/-f "
26200 PRINT ""
26250 PRINT "  FOR THIS CASE Xo IS 1.5 TIMES f, OR"
26300 PRINT "            Xo=1.5f "
26350 PRINT ""
26400 PRINT "     Xi = -0.75f, VIRTUAL IMAGE!!"
26450 PRINT ""
26500 PRINT "    THE MAGNIFICATION IS -Xi/Xo, OR"
26550 PRINT "           MAG = 1/2"
26600 PRINT ""
26650 PRINT " MAG IS POSITIVE, HENCE AN ERECT IMAGE"
26700 PRINT ""
26750 PRINT " -f IS USED IN THE THIN LENS EQUATION"
26800 PRINT " BECAUSE A NEGATIVE THIN LENS HAS A"
26850 PRINT "     NEGATIVE FOCAL LENGTH"
26900 'BB=25: GOSUB 6750
26950 A$=INKEY$: IF A$="" THEN 26950
27000 LOCATE 25,1
```

```
27050 PRINT ""
27100 CLS
27150 GOSUB 42050
27200 LINE (272,95)-(272,105),2 'back 2f
27250 LINE (142,95)-(142,105),2 'forward 2f
27300 LINE (159,100)-(159,70),1 'object
27350 LINE (159,70)-(163,75),1 'arrow point
27400 LINE (159,70)-(155,75),1 'arrow point
27450 PRINT "object ray appears to come from infinity as it hits
      the lens"
27500 BB=5: GOSUB 41300
27550 LINE (159,70)-(208,70) 'hori. trac
27600 PRINT "the lens forces this ray to diverge as if it came from
      the front focus"
27650 BB=5: GOSUB 41300
27700 PRINT "next a ray from the object passes through the
      vertex"
27750 LINE (176,100)-(249,30) 'focus tra
27800 BB=5: GOSUB 41300
27850 LINE (159,70)-(229,113) 'vertex
27900 BB=5: GOSUB 41300
27950 FOR I=1 TO 8
28000 PRINT ""
28050 NEXT I
28100 LINE (189,100)-(189,88),2 'image
28150 CIRCLE (189,88),10,2,,,1
28200 PRINT "the image is minified"
28250 PRINT "erect and virtual"
28300 PRINT ""
28350 PRINT "NOTE: THE VIRTUAL"
28400 PRINT "IMAGE IS ALWAYS BETWEEN"
28450 PRINT "THE FRONT FOCUS AND THE"
28500 PRINT "LENS FOR A NEGATIVE LENS"
28550 LOCATE 25,1
28600 PRINT "HIT SPACE BAR TO MOVE ON"
28650 A$=INKEY$: IF A$="" THEN 28650
28700 'BB=15: GOSUB 7450
28750 CLS
28800 IF ANS=0 THEN GOTO 4650
28850 '******* THIS IS EXAMPLE #8 ********
28900 CLS
```

```
28950 LOCATE 25,1
29000 PRINT "HIT SPACE BAR TO MOVE ON"
29050 PRINT ""
29100 PRINT "   **THIS IS A TWO LENS EXAMPLE**"
29150 PRINT""
29200 PRINT "THE OBJECT IS SEVERAL FOCAL LENGTHS
  FROM THE FRONT LENS"
29250 PRINT "NOTE THAT THE IMAGE WILL BE MINIMIZED
  AND ERECT"
29300 PRINT""
29350 PRINT"      ***********"
29400 PRINT " TO AVOID CONFUSION, TRACE REAL RAYS"
29450 PRINT "THROUGH THE SYSTEM.  TRACE RAYS
  THROUGH"
29500 PRINT " THE FIRST LENS AS BEFORE TO SHOW THE"
29550 PRINT "DIRECTION RAYS MUST GO AS THEY AP-
  PROACH"
29600 PRINT " THE SECOND LENS.  THEN USE RAYS WHICH"
29650 PRINT " APPROACH THE NEXT LENS FROM USABLE"
29700 PRINT " DIRECTIONS.  THE BEST DIRECTIONS ARE  "
29750 PRINT "  PARALLEL TO THE OPTICAL AXIS AND"
29800 PRINT "THROUGH THE VERTEX.  "
29850 PRINT "      ***********"
29900 PRINT ""
29950 PRINT ""
30000 PRINT ""
30050 'BB=27: GOSUB 6750
30100 A$=INKEY$: IF A$="" THEN 30100
30150 LOCATE 25,1
30200 PRINT ""
30250 CLS
30300 GOSUB 42650
30350 LINE (0,100)-(0,70),1 'object
30400 LINE (0,70)-(3,75),1 'arrow point
30450 PRINT "Begin the ray trace as before."
30500  BB=5: GOSUB 41300
30550 PRINT ""
30600 LINE (0,70)-(178,70) 'hori. trace
30650 LINE (178,70)-(264,150) 'focus trac
30700 LINE (0,70)-(272,116) 'vertex
30750 BB=5: GOSUB 41300
```

```
30800 PRINT "The image is used to show the direction which the
   rays take through the first lens on their way to the next lens."
30850 BB=8: GOSUB 41300
30900 LINE (218,100)-(218,107),2 'image
30950 CIRCLE (218,107),5,2,,,1
31000 BB=5: GOSUB 41300
31050 FOR I=1 TO 8
31100 PRINT ""
31150 NEXT I
31200 PRINT "Now choose a ray"
31250 PRINT "which goes through"
31300 PRINT "lens 1 and passes"
31350 PRINT "in the image direction"
31400 PRINT "parallel to the axis."
31450 LINE (218,107)-(253,107),2,,&HCCCC 'hori.,lens 2
31500 LINE (253,107)-(350,71),2 'focus trace,lens 2
31550 BB=5: GOSUB 41300
31600 PRINT "***"
31650 PRINT "Now choose a ray"
31700 PRINT "which goes through lens"
31750 PRINT "1 and passes in the image direction"
31800 PRINT "headed to the vertex."
31850 LINE (218,107)-(350,81),2 'vertex,lens 2
31900 CIRCLE (295,92),5,1,,,1 'final
31950 LINE (295,100)-(295,93),2 'image
32000 LOCATE 25,1
32050 PRINT "HIT SPACE BAR TO MOVE ON"
32100 A$=INKEY$: IF A$="" THEN 32100
32150 'BB=15: GOSUB 7450
32200 CLS
32250 IF ANS=0 THEN GOTO 4650
32300 '******** THIS IS EXAMPLE #9 ********
32350 CLS
32400 LOCATE 25,1
32450 PRINT "HIT SPACE BAR TO MOVE ON"
32500 PRINT ""
32550 PRINT "  **THIS IS A TWO LENS EXAMPLE, #2**"
32600 PRINT""
32650 PRINT "THE OBJECT IS SEVERAL FOCAL LENGTHS
   FROM THE FRONT LENS"
32700 PRINT "NOTE THAT THE IMAGE WILL BE MINIMIZED,
```

```
     REAL, AND INVERTED"
32750 PRINT""
32800 PRINT"          ************"
32850 PRINT " TO AVOID CONFUSION, TRACE REAL RAYS"
32900 PRINT "THROUGH THE SYSTEM.  TRACE RAYS
     THROUGH"
32950 PRINT " THE FIRST LENS AS BEFORE TO SHOW THE"
33000 PRINT "DIRECTION RAYS MUST GO AS THEY AP-
     PROACH"
33050 PRINT " THE SECOND LENS.  THEN USE RAYS WHICH"
33100 PRINT " APPROACH THE NEXT LENS FROM USABLE"
33150 PRINT " DIRECTIONS.  THE BEST DIRECTIONS ARE  "
33200 PRINT "   PARALLEL TO THE OPTICAL AXIS AND"
33250 PRINT "THROUGH THE VERTEX.  "
33300 PRINT"          ************"
33350 PRINT ""
33400 PRINT ""
33450 PRINT ""
33500 'BB=25: GOSUB 6750
33550 A$=INKEY$: IF A$="" THEN 33550
33600 LOCATE 25,1
33650 PRINT ""
33700 CLS
33750 GOSUB 43400
33800 LINE (0,100)-(0,70),1 'object
33850 LINE (0,70)-(3,75),1 'arrow point
33900 PRINT "Begin the ray trace as before."
33950  BB=5: GOSUB 41300
34000 PRINT ""
34050 LINE (0,70)-(178,70) 'hori. trace
34100 LINE (178,70)-(298,150) 'focus trac
34150 LINE (0,70)-(272,116) 'vertex
34200 BB=5: GOSUB 41300
34250 PRINT "The image is used to show the direction which the
     rays take through the first lens on their way to the next lens."
34300 BB=8: GOSUB 41300
34350 LINE (239,100)-(239,111),2 'image
34400 CIRCLE (239,111),5,2,,,1
34450 BB=5: GOSUB 41300
34500 FOR I=1 TO 8
34550 PRINT ""
```

```
34600 NEXT I
34650 PRINT "Now choose a ray"
34700 PRINT "which goes through"
34750 PRINT "lens 1 and passes"
34800 PRINT "in the image direction"
34850 PRINT "parallel to the axis."
34900 LINE (178,111)-(239,111),2,,&HCCCC 'hori.,lens 2
34950 LINE (210,111)-(350,49),2 'focus trace,lens 2
35000 BB=7: GOSUB 41300
35050 PRINT "***"
35100 PRINT "Now choose a ray"
35150 PRINT "which goes through lens"
35200 PRINT "1 and passes in the image direction"
35250 PRINT "headed to the vertex."
35300 LINE (178,88)-(350,150),2 'vertex,lens 2
35350 CIRCLE (225,105),5,1,,,1 'final
35400 LINE (225,100)-(225,105),2 'image
35450 LOCATE 25,1
35500 PRINT "HIT SPACE BAR TO MOVE ON"
35550 A$=INKEY$: IF A$="" THEN 35550
35600 'BB=15: GOSUB 7450
35650 CLS
35700 IF ANS=0 THEN GOTO 4650
35750 '******** THIS IS EXAMPLE #10 ********
35800 CLS
35850 LOCATE 25,1
35900 PRINT "HIT SPACE BAR TO MOVE ON"
35950 PRINT ""
36000 PRINT "**THIS IS A TWO LENS EXAMPLE, WITH A
      NEGATIVE LENS**"
36050 PRINT ""
36100 PRINT "THE OBJECT IS SEVERAL FOCAL LENGTHS
      FROM THE FRONT LENS"
36150 PRINT "NOTE THAT THE IMAGE WILL BE VIRTUAL
      AND ERECT"
36200 PRINT""
36250 PRINT"          ************"
36300 PRINT " TO AVOID CONFUSION, TRACE REAL RAYS"
36350 PRINT "THROUGH THE SYSTEM.  TRACE RAYS
      THROUGH"
36400 PRINT " THE FIRST LENS AS BEFORE TO SHOW THE"
```

```
36450 PRINT "DIRECTION RAYS MUST GO AS THEY AP-
  PROACH"
36500 PRINT " THE SECOND LENS. THEN USE RAYS WHICH"
36550 PRINT " APPROACH THE NEXT LENS FROM USABLE"
36600 PRINT " DIRECTIONS.  THE BEST DIRECTIONS ARE  "
36650 PRINT "   PARALLEL TO THE OPTICAL AXIS AND"
36700 PRINT "THROUGH THE VERTEX.  "
36750 PRINT"        ************"
36800 PRINT""
36850 PRINT""
36900 'BB=25: GOSUB 6750
36950 A$=INKEY$: IF A$="" THEN 36950
37000 LOCATE 25,1
37050 PRINT ""
37100 CLS
37150 GOSUB 44150
37200 LINE (0,100)-(0,70),1 'object
37250 LINE (0,70)-(3,75),1 'arrow point
37300 PRINT "Begin the ray trace as before."
37350  BB=5: GOSUB 41300
37400 PRINT ""
37450 LINE (0,70)-(178,70) 'hori. trace
37500 LINE (178,70)-(298,150) 'focus trac
37550 LINE (0,70)-(272,116) 'vertex
37600 BB=5: GOSUB 41300
37650 PRINT "The image is used to show the direction which the
  rays take through the first lens on their way to the next lens."
37700 BB=8: GOSUB 41300
37750 LINE (239,100)-(239,111),2 'image
37800 CIRCLE (239,111),5,2,,,1
37850 BB=5: GOSUB 41300
37900 FOR I=1 TO 8
37950 PRINT ""
38000 NEXT I
38050 PRINT "Now choose a ray"
38100 PRINT "which goes through"
38150 PRINT "lens 1 and passes"
38200 PRINT "in the image direction"
38250 PRINT "parallel to the axis."
38300 LINE (178,111)-(239,111),2,,&HCCCC 'hori.,lens 2
38350 LINE (20,30)-(208,111),2 'focus trace,lens 2
```

```
38400 BB=7: GOSUB 41300
38450 PRINT "***"
38500 PRINT "Now choose a ray"
38550 PRINT "which goes through lens"
38600 PRINT "1 and passes in the image direction"
38650 PRINT "headed to the vertex."
38700 LINE (40,46)-(350,146),2 'vertex,lens 2
38750 CIRCLE (115,70),5,1,,,1  'final
38800 LINE (115,100)-(115,70),2 'image
38850 LOCATE 25,1
38900 PRINT "HIT SPACE BAR TO MOVE ON"
38950 A$=INKEY$: IF A$="" THEN 38950
39000 'BB=15: GOSUB 7450
39050 CLS
39100 IF ANS=0 THEN GOTO 4650
39150 CLS
39200 LOCATE 25,1
39250 PRINT "HIT SPACE BAR TO MOVE ON"
39300 PRINT ""
39350 PRINT "  **THIS IS A FIELD OF VIEW EXAMPLE**"
39351 PRINT ""
39352 PRINT "A SIMPLE ROUTINE IS PRESENTED FOR A "
39353 PRINT "TWO LENS SYSTEM.  AS IS TRUE OF ALL "
39354 PRINT "THE EXAMPLES IN THIS TUTORIAL, MORE"
39355 PRINT "COMPLICATED SYSTEMS SHOULD BE STUD-
   IED "
39356 PRINT "WITH THE MATHEMATICAL REPRESENTA-
   TION. "
39357 PRINT "THESE EXAMPLES HELP UNDERSTAND THE
   "
39358 PRINT "BASIC PRINCIPLES BEHIND THE OPTICS,"
39359 PRINT "IN THIS EXAMPLE, GIVEN AN OBJECT
   PLANE,"
39360 PRINT "THE MAXIMUM OBJECT SIZE IS FOUND. "
39361 PRINT "*************************************"
39362 PRINT""
39363 PRINT "THERE ARE FOUR BASIC STEPS TO THE "
39364 PRINT "PROBLEM. "
39365 PRINT "1. CHOOSE THE OBJECT PLANE."
39366 PRINT "3  DRAW EXCLUSION ZONE."
39367 PRINT "2. FIND THE FIRST IMAGE."
```

```
39368 PRINT "4. TRACE BACK TO MAX OBJECT SIZE."
39369 PRINT""
39370 A$=INKEY$: IF A$="" THEN 39370
39371 CLS
39372 LOCATE 25,1
39373 PRINT "HIT SPACE BAR TO MOVE ON"
39374 PRINT "THIS LENS SYSTEM HAS ONE FINAL IMAGE"
39375 PRINT "PLANE.  IF YOU USE YOUR EYE, THEN "
39376 PRINT "INCLUDE IT AS THE FINAL LENS.    "
39377 PRINT "WHEN YOU MOVE YOUR EYE WHILE LOOK-
      ING"
39378 PRINT "THROUGH A LENS SYSTEM THE FIELD OF
      VIEW"
39379 PRINT "CHANGES.  THIS MUST BE TAKEN INTO "
39380 PRINT "ACCOUNT. "
39381 PRINT""
39382 PRINT"**********************************"
39383 PRINT""
39384 PRINT "THIS APPROACH CAN BE USED FOR MORE"
39385 PRINT "LENSES.  CONTINUE FORMING IMAGES AND"
39386 PRINT "FIND THE LENS, OR STOP, THAT RESTRICTS"
39387 PRINT "RAYS FROM GETTING THROUGH THE SYS-
      TEM."
39388 PRINT "OF COURSE, THIS IS THE FIELD STOP FOR"
39389 PRINT "THE SYSTEM.  MATHEMATICALLY, THIS IS"
39390 PRINT "THE SAME AS FINDING THE IMAGE OF THE"
39391 PRINT "FIELD STOP IN THE OBJECT AND IMAGE"
39392 PRINT "DIRECTIONS.  THE SAME PROCEDURE IS"
39393 PRINT "USED WITH THE APERTURE STOP TO FIND"
39394 PRINT "THE PUPILS.  HERE YOU ARE FINDING THE"
39395 PRINT "*** ENTRANCE AND EXIT WINDOWS ***.
39400 PRINT""
39450 A$=INKEY$: IF A$="" THEN 39450
39500 CLS
39550 GOSUB 45000
39570 PRINT "1. Choose obj. plane"
39571 PRINT "Ray trace as before(pick any obj. size)"
39575  BB=3: GOSUB 41300
39600 LINE (80,130)-(80,100),1 'object
39650 LINE (80,100)-(83,105),1 'arrow point
39700 LINE (80,100)-(77,105),1 'arrow point
```

```
39800  BB=2: GOSUB 41300
39805 PRINT "2. Find first image.
39850 LINE (80,100)-(178,100) 'hori. trace
39900 LINE (178,100)-(265,160) 'focus
39950 LINE (80,100)-(280,161) 'vertex
40000 BB=3: GOSUB 41300
40050 LINE (255,130)-(255,154),2 'image
40100 CIRCLE (255,154),5,2,,,1
40150 BB=3: GOSUB 41300
40175 LINE (80,130)-(80,1),1,,&HCCCC 'object
40200 LINE (255,130)-(255,190),2,,&HCCCC 'image line
40240 PRINT "3. Find exclusion zone.
40250 LINE (178,100)-(260,191),1,,&HCCCC 'exclusion line #1
40298 LINE (178,160)-(255,185),1,,&HCCCC 'exclusion line #2
40299 BB=3: GOSUB 41300
40300 PRINT "4. Trace back to max obj. size."
40301 FOR I=1 TO 12
40302 PRINT ""
40303 NEXT I
40304 PRINT "The exclusion zone"
40305 PRINT "is defined by an"
40306 PRINT "object whose rays"
40307 PRINT "get through lens 1"
40308 PRINT "but none from this"
40309 PRINT "object point can  "
40310 PRINT "get to lens 2"
40315 BB=5: GOSUB 41300
40350 LINE (60,41)-(258,179),1,,&HCCCC 'back to the object plane
40400 LINE (70,55)-(20,55),1 'new object size
40450 LINE (70,55)-(67,52),1 'arrow
40500 LINE (70,55)-(67,58),1 'arrow
40550 'LINE (178,152)-(239,152),2,,&HCCCC 'hori.,lens 2
40600 'LINE (235,152)-(290,100),2 'focus trace,lens 2
40650 BB=5: GOSUB 41300
40655 PRINT "                Final max. image"
40656 BB=2: GOSUB 41300
40700 'LINE (230,127)-(300,200),2 'vertex,lens 2
40750 CIRCLE (245,142),5,1,,,1 'final
40800 LINE (245,115)-(245,142),2 'image
40850 LOCATE 25,1
40900 PRINT "HIT SPACE BAR TO MOVE ON"
```

```
40950 A$=INKEY$: IF A$="" THEN 40950
41000 CLS
41050 IF ANS=0 THEN GOTO 4650
41100 END
41150 '
41200 'TIME DELAY SUBROUTINE
41250 '
41300 A=TIMER+(BB*SPEED)
41350 B=TIMER
41400 IF B>A THEN 41500
41450 GOTO 41350
41500 RETURN
41550 '
41600 'BASIC THIN LENS WITH AXIS
41650 '
41700 CIRCLE (351,100),150,,.9*PI,1.1*PI,1
41750 CIRCLE (65,100),150,,1.9*PI,.1*PI,1
41800 LINE (208,20)-(208,180) 'vertical
41850 LINE(0,100)-(320,100) 'horizontal
41900 LINE (240,95)-(240,105),2 'back focus
41950 LINE (176,95)-(176,105),2 'front focus
42000 RETURN
42050 '
42100 'BASIC THIN LENS WITH AXIS(negative lens)
42150 '
42200 CIRCLE (363,100),150,,.9*PI,1.1*PI,1
42250 CIRCLE (53,100),150,,1.9*PI,.1*PI,1
42300 LINE (208,20)-(208,180) 'vertical
42350 LINE(0,100)-(320,100) 'horizontal
42400 LINE(198,58)-(218,58) 'horizontal
42450 LINE(198,142)-(218,142) 'horizontal
42500 LINE (240,95)-(240,105),2 'back focus
42550 LINE (176,95)-(176,105),2 'front focus
42600 RETURN
42650 '
42700 'TWO LENS SYSTEM WITH AXIS
42750 '
42800 CIRCLE (396,100),150,,.9*PI,1.1*PI,1
42850 CIRCLE (321,100),150,,.9*PI,1.1*PI,1
42900 CIRCLE (110,100),150,,1.9*PI,.1*PI,1
42950 CIRCLE (35,100),150,,1.9*PI,.1*PI,1
```

```
43000 LINE (253,20)-(253,180) 'vertical
43050 LINE (178,20)-(178,180) 'vertical
43100 LINE(0,100)-(320,100) 'horizontal
43150 LINE (275,95)-(275,105),2 'back focus
43200 LINE (210,93)-(210,107),2 'back focus
43250 LINE (231,95)-(231,105),2 'front focus
43300 LINE (146,93)-(146,107),2 'front focus
43350 RETURN
43400 '
43450 'TWO LENS SYSTEM WITH AXIS #2
43500 '
43550 CIRCLE (353,100),150,,.9*PI,1.1*PI,1
43600 CIRCLE (321,100),150,,.9*PI,1.1*PI,1
43650 CIRCLE (66,100),150,,1.9*PI,.1*PI,1
43700 CIRCLE (34,100),150,,1.9*PI,.1*PI,1
43750 LINE (210,20)-(210,180) 'vertical
43800 LINE (178,20)-(178,180) 'vertical
43850 LINE(0,100)-(320,100) 'horizontal
43900 LINE (235,95)-(235,105),2 'back focus
43950 LINE (223,93)-(223,107),2 'back focus
44000 LINE (185,95)-(185,105),2 'front focus
44050 LINE (133,93)-(133,107),2 'front focus
44100 RETURN
44150 '
44200 'TWO LENS SYSTEM WITH NEGATIVE LENS
44250 '
44300 CIRCLE (363,100),150,,.9*PI,1.1*PI,1 'POS. LENS
44350 CIRCLE (321,100),150,,.9*PI,1.1*PI,1
44400 CIRCLE (53,100),150,,1.9*PI,.1*PI,1  'POS. LENS
44450 CIRCLE (34,100),150,,1.9*PI,.1*PI,1
44500 LINE (178,20)-(178,180) 'vertical
44550 LINE (208,20)-(208,180) 'vertical
44600 LINE(0,100)-(320,100) 'horizontal
44650 LINE(198,58)-(218,58) 'horizontal
44700 LINE (223,93)-(223,107),2 'back focus
44750 LINE (133,93)-(133,107),2 'front focus
44800 LINE(198,142)-(218,142) 'horizontal
44850 LINE (235,95)-(235,105),2 'back focus
44900 LINE (181,95)-(181,105),2 'front focus
44950 RETURN
```

```
45000 '
45050 'TWO LENS SYSTEM WITH AXIS #2 (FIELD OF VIEW)
45100 '
45150 CIRCLE (380,130),150,,.93*PI,1.07*PI,1
45200 CIRCLE (324,130),150,,.93*PI,1.07*PI,1
45250 CIRCLE (88,130),150,,1.93*PI,.07*PI,1
45300 CIRCLE (32,130),150,,1.93*PI,.07*PI,1
45350 LINE (234,50)-(234,190) 'vertical
45400 LINE (178,50)-(178,190) 'vertical
45450 LINE(0,130)-(320,130) 'horizontal
45500 LINE (259,125)-(259,135),2 'back focus
45550 LINE (223,123)-(223,137),2 'back focus
45600 LINE (209,125)-(209,135),2 'front focus
45650 LINE (133,123)-(133,137),2 'front focus
45700 RETURN
45750
      '*********************************************************************
45800
      '*********************************************************************
45850 'THIS IS PROGRAM LENS. A LENS SYSTEM OF THIN
      LENSES IS ANALYZED IN
45900 'THIS PROGRAM.
45950 CLS:'CALL BAS87
46000 DEFDBL A-H,O-Z
46050 DIM
      ALENS(5,2,2),FL(5),DIS(4),DIA(5),TR(5,2,2),QQ(2,2),ANGLE(5),OPP(
      5)
46100 DIM AD(5)
46150 PRINT "INPUT A TITLE OR PHRASE TO DESCRIBE THE
      OUTPUT"
46200 INPUT B$
46250 PRINT
      "*********************************************************** "
46300 PRINT B$
46350 INPUT "NUMBER OF OBJECTS ",NLENS
46400 PRINT " "
46450 PRINT " "
46500 PRINT "***ALL LENGTHS NEED TO BE IN CENTIME-
      TERS***"
46550 PRINT " "
46600 IF NLENS=1 THEN GOTO 54200
```

```
46650 INPUT"ARE THERE ANY NON-IMAGING STOPS IN THE
    SYSTEM? (NO, YES) ",STOPS$
46700 IF STOPS$="no" THEN STOPS$="NO"
46750 IF STOPS$="n" THEN STOPS$="NO"
46800 IF STOPS$="N" THEN STOPS$="NO"
46850 IF STOPS$="Y" THEN STOPS$="YES"
46900 IF STOPS$="y" THEN STOPS$="YES"
46950 PRINT " "
47000 IF STOPS$="yes" THEN STOPS$="YES"
47050 FOR I=1 TO NLENS
47100  IF STOPS$="YES" THEN PRINT "IS OBJECT(";I;") A
    STOP? (NO, YES) "
47150  IF STOPS$="YES" THEN INPUT STP$
47200 IF STP$="no" THEN STP$="NO"
47250 IF STP$="n" THEN STP$="NO"
47300 IF STP$="N" THEN STP$="NO"
47350 IF STP$="y" THEN STP$="YES"
47400 IF STP$="yes" THEN STP$="YES"
47450 IF STP$="Y" THEN STP$="YES"
47500  IF STP$="YES" THEN FL(I)=999999999999999#
47550  IF STP$="YES" THEN GOTO 47700
47600 PRINT "INPUT THE FOCAL LENGTH FOR OBJECT(";I;")"
47650 INPUT FL(I)
47700 PRINT "INPUT THE DIAMETER FOR OBJECT(";I;")"
47750 INPUT DIA(I)
47800 NEXT I
47850 NN=NLENS-1
47900 FOR I=1 TO NN
47950 PRINT "INPUT THE DISTANCE BETWEEN OBJECT(";I;")
    AND OBJECT(";I+1;")"
48000 INPUT DIS(I)
48050 NEXT I
48100 INPUT "INPUT DISTANCE FROM FIRST LENS (OR
    OBJECT) TO OBJECT BEING IMAGED ",DOBJ
48150 PRINT " "
48200 PRINT " "
48250 PRINT
    "*****************************************************************"
48300 PRINT B$
48350 PRINT " "
```

```
48400 FOR I=1 TO NLENS
48450 ALENS(I,1,1)=1      'LENS MATRIX
48500 ALENS(I,2,1)=0
48550 ALENS(I,2,2)=1
48600 ALENS(I,1,2)=-(1/FL(I))
48650 TR(I,1,1)=1         'TRANSFER MATRIX
48700 TR(I,1,2)=0
48750 IF I = 1 THEN TR(I,2,1)=DOBJ ELSE TR(I,2,1)=DIS(I-1)
48800 TR(I,2,2)=1
48850 NEXT I
48900 'NOW CALCULATE THE SYSTEM MATRIX
48950 GOSUB 54900
49000 PRINT " "
49050 PRINT "THE SYSTEM MATRIX IS"
49100 PRINT USING "A(1,1)=###.#####
  A(1,2)=###.#####";QQ(1,1),QQ(1,2)
49150 PRINT USING "A(2,1)=###.#####
  A(2,2)=###.#####";QQ(2,1),QQ(2,2)
49155 IF QQ(1,2)=0 THEN PRINT "THE EFFECTIVE FOCAL
  LENGTH IS** INFINITE **"
49156 IF QQ(1,2)=0 THEN PRINT "THE IMAGE IS AT INFIN-
  ITY"
49157 IF QQ(1,2)=0 THEN PRINT "THE OBJECT IS IMAGED AT
  INFINITY"
49158 IF QQ(1,2)=0 THEN GOTO 54850
49200 EFOC=-1/QQ(1,2)
49250 PRINT USING "THE EFFECTIVE FOCAL LENGTH IS
  EFOC=####.### CM";EFOC
49300 V1H1=(1-QQ(1,1))/(-QQ(1,2))
49350 V2H2=(QQ(2,2)-1)/(-QQ(1,2))
49400 PRINT " "
49450 PRINT "***** THE PRINCIPAL PLANES FOR THE SYS-
  TEM *****"
49500 IF V1H1>0 THEN PRINT USING "THE FIRST PRINCIPAL
  PLANE IS ####.## CM TO THE RIGHT SIDE OF THE FIRST
  VERTEX";ABS(V1H1)
49550 IF V1H1<0 THEN PRINT USING "THE FIRST PRINCIPAL
  PLANE IS ####.## CM TO THE LEFT SIDE OF THE FIRST
  VERTEX";ABS(V1H1)
49600 IF V2H2>0 THEN PRINT USING "THE SECOND PRINCI-
  PAL PLANE IS ####.## CM TO THE RIGHT SIDE OF THE
```

LAST VERTEX";ABS(V2H2)

49650 IF V2H2<0 THEN PRINT USING "THE SECOND PRINCI-
PAL PLANE IS ####.## CM TO THE LEFT SIDE OF THE LAST
VERTEX";ABS(V2H2)

49700 SO=DOBJ+V1H1

49750 SI=EFOC*SO/(SO-EFOC)

49800 PRINT USING "THE OBJECT DISTANCE IS So=#####.##
CM (FROM 1ST PRINCIPAL PLANE)";SO

49850 PRINT USING "THE IMAGE DISTANCE IS Si=#####.##
CM (FROM 2ND PRINCIPAL PLANE)";SI

49900 PRINT " "

49950 PRINT " "

50000 'NOW CALCULATE ENTRANCE AND EXIT PUPIL

50050 DIS1=0!

50100 NNN=NLENS-1

50150 NNN2=NNN

50200 NNN1=NLENS+1

50250 NLENS1=NLENS

50300 FOR K=1 TO NNN2

50350 FOR J=1 TO NNN

50400 DIS1=DIS1+DIS(J)

50450 NEXT J

50500 SI1=0!

50550 DIA1=0!

50600 DIA1=DIA(NLENS1)

50650 ' THE FOLLOWING LOOP FINDS THE IMAGE OF ONE
LENS THROUGH THE PRECEDING LENSES

50700 PRINT " SO   SI   AMT   ADJ   OP   OBJECT"

50750 FOR I=1 TO NNN

50800 SO1=SI1+DIS(NLENS1-I) 'DISTANCE FROM OBJ. TO
IMAGING LENS

50850 SO1=-SO1

50900 DIS1=DIS1-DIS(NLENS1-I)

50950 AFL=FL(NLENS1-I) 'FOCAL LENGTH OF IMAGING
LENS

51000 AFL=-AFL

51050 SI1=AFL*SO1/(SO1-AFL) 'IMAGE DIS. OF OBJ.

51100 AMT=ABS(SI1/SO1) 'MAGNIFICATION

51150 ADJ=DOBJ+SI1+DIS1 'ADJACENT SIDE OF TRIANGLE
FOR CALCULATING PUPIL ANG.

51200 OP=DIA1/2*AMT 'OPPOSITE SIDE OF TRIANGLE

```
51250 DIA1=2*OP
51300 PRINT USING"#.####^^^^  #.####^^^^ #.####^^^^ #.
   ####^^^^ #.####^^^^ ###";SO1,SI1,AMT,ADJ,OP,(NLENS+1-K)
51350 NEXT I
51400 ' ANG IS THE CONE ANGLE OF THE LENS IMAGE
   AFTER PASSING THROUGH
51450 ' EACH LENS NECESSARY TO FIND THE PUPIL
51500 ANG=ATN(OP/ADJ)
51550 IF ADJ<DOBJ THEN ANG=10
51600 NNN=NNN-1
51650 NNN1=NNN1-1
51700 NLENS1=NLENS1-1
51750 ANGLE(NLENS+1-K)=ANG
51800 OPP(K+1)=OP
51850 AD(K+1)=ADJ
51900 NEXT K
51950 OP=DIA(1)/2
52000 ANG=ATN(OP/DOBJ)
52050 ANGLE(1)=ANG
52100 PANG=ANGLE(1)
52150  OP1=2*OP
52200 ADJ1=DOBJ
52250 AINT=1
52300 ' PANG IS THE PUPIL ANGLE IN RADIANS
52350 FOR I=2 TO NLENS
52400 IF ANGLE(I)<PANG THEN AINT=I
52450 IF ANGLE(I)<PANG THEN OP1=OPP(NLENS-I+2)*2
52500 IF ANGLE(I)<PANG THEN ADJ1=AD(NLENS-I+2)
52550 IF ANGLE(I)<PANG THEN PANG=ANGLE(I)
52603 PRINT " "
52605 PRINT "** HIT SPACE BAR TO MOVE ON **"
52610 A$=INKEY$: IF A$="" THEN 52610
52600 NEXT I
52650 PRINT " "
52700 PRINT"*********** ENTRANCE PUPIL ***************"
52750 PRINT USING" THE APERTURE STOP IS OBJECT
   ###";AINT
52800 DI=ADJ1
52850 PRINT USING " THE DIAMETER OF THE PUPIL IS
   ###.### CM AND IT IS LOCATED #.###^^^^ CM FROM THE
   OBJECT, WITH AN ANGLE OF #.####^^^^
```

```
   RAD";OP1,DI,2*PANG
52900 PRINT " "
52950 PRINT"**************** EXIT PUPIL ******************"
53000 II=1
53050 DIS1=0
53100 ADJ2=SI+V2H2
53150 IF AINT>NNN2 THEN GOTO 53800
53200 DIA1=DIA(AINT)
53250 SI1=0
53300 FOR I=AINT TO NNN2
53350 SO1=DIS(I)-SI1
53400 AFL=FL(I+1)
53405 BCB=SO1-AFL
53406 IF BCB=0 THEN BCB=9.999999E-20
53450 SI1=AFL*SO1/(SO1-AFL)
53500 AMT=ABS(SI1/SO1)
53550 OP=DIA1*AMT/2
53600 DIA1=2*OP
53650 NEXT I
53700 ADJ=ADJ2-SI1
53750 ANG=ATN(OP/ADJ)
53800 IF AINT>NNN2 THEN ANG=ATN((DIA(NLENS)/2)/ADJ2)
53850 PRINT USING" THE APERTURE STOP IS OBJECT
  ###";AINT
53900 OP1=2*OP
53950 DI=ADJ
54000 IF AINT>NNN2 THEN OP1=DIA(NLENS)
54050 IF AINT>NNN2 THEN DI=ADJ2
54100 PRINT USING " THE DIAMETER OF THE PUPIL IS
  ###.### CM AND IT IS LOCATED #.###^^^^ CM FROM THE
  IMAGE,  WITH AN ANGLE OF #.####^^^^RAD";OP1,DI,2*ANG
54150 GOTO 54850
54200 INPUT "INPUT FOCAL LENGTH ";F
54250 INPUT "INPUT DISTANCE TO OBJECT ";SO
54300 SI=1/(1/F-1/SO)
54350 PRINT ""
54400 PRINT USING " THE FOCAL LENGTH IS = ###.### CM";F
54450 PRINT USING " THE OBJECT IS LOCATED ####.### CM
  FROM THE LENS";SO
54500 PRINT USING " THE IMAGE IS LOCATED ####.### CM
  FROM THE LENS";SI
```

```
54550 PRINT "**** POSITIVE- TO THE RIGHT, NEGATIVE TO
  THE LEFT****"
54600 PRINT ""
54650 M=-SI/SO
54700 PRINT USING " THE MAGNIFICATION IS ####.###";M
54750 IF M<0 THEN PRINT "THEREFORE, THE IMAGE IS
  INVERTED"
54800 IF M>0 THEN PRINT "THEREFORE, THE IMAGE IS
  ERECT"
54850 END
54900 REM THIS SUBROUTINE CALCULATES THE SYSTEM
  MATRIX.
54950 QSUM=0
55000 FOR I=1 TO 2
55050 FOR II=1 TO 2
55100 FOR J=1 TO 2
55150 QSUM=QSUM+ALENS(NLENS,I,J)*TR(NLENS,J,II)
55200 NEXT J
55250 QQ(I,II)=QSUM
55300 QSUM=0
55350 NEXT II
55400 NEXT I
55450 ICOUNT=0
55500 NN1=2*(NLENS-1)-1
55550 JJ1=NLENS
55600 JJ2=NLENS
55650 FOR JJ=1 TO NN1
55700 ICOUNT=ICOUNT+1
55750 IF ICOUNT=1 THEN JJ1=JJ1-1
55800 IF ICOUNT=2 THEN JJ2=JJ2-1
55850 QSUM=0
55900 FOR I=1 TO 2
55950 FOR II=1 TO 2
56000 FOR J=1 TO 2
56050 IF ICOUNT=1 THEN
  QSUM=QSUM+QQ(I,J)*ALENS(JJ1,J,II)
56100 IF ICOUNT=2 THEN QSUM=QSUM+QQ(I,J)*TR(JJ2,J,II)
56150 NEXT J
56200 QQ(I,II)=QSUM
56250 QSUM=0
56300 NEXT II
```

```
56350 NEXT I
56400 IF ICOUNT=2 THEN ICOUNT=0
56450 'PRINT QQ(1,1),QQ(1,2),QQ(2,1),QQ(2,2)
56500 NEXT JJ
56550 RETURN
```

INDEX

UV, 18
UV Absorption of the Eye, 18

V
visible, 18
vitreous, 3, 6, 10, 11, 57
vitreous humor, 10

W
welder's flash, 5